Anti-Aging & Health Benefits of Sex

Dr. Shelley

For MATT!
Appreciate your guest!
Thankyou for doing what
you're doing

DR. Shelley

March 8, 2022

Dr. Shelley's LLC
6130 W. Flamingo Rd. 707
Las Vegas, NV 89103, USA
www.DrShelleys.com

ISBN: 1490947051
ISBN-13: 987-1490947051

Thank you to everyone who helped me with my dissertation.

My appreciation goes to Denie for understanding how important it was for me to do this and to encourage me, even though you lost you "secretary" during that time – now you have one with a PhD!!

Thank you to Dr. Keith and Dr. Victoria for your advice and guidance.

Thank you to my special friends for helping me with my statistical analysis and graphs and to Nicole for your editing expertise.

And a special thank you to all the *"swingers"* who took the time to fill out the questionnaire for my research project.

I dedicate this dissertation to all the wonderful individuals and couples I have worked with over the years who inspired me to pursue further studies in this fascinating field. Thank you for allowing me to be part of your lives and to experience how truly beneficial positive sexual experiences are for health and well-being.

CONTENTS

ABSTRACT

Outlined are specific health benefits associated with sex and other sexual activity, including references to the *Anti-Aging Benefits of Sex* – how sex can help the individual stay young, and keep relationships vibrant and alive. This research was aimed primarily at heterosexual partnering and focuses predominantly on the anti-aging and health benefits of penile-vaginal-intercourse (PVI). Research shows that along with physical health benefits associated with this type of sexual activity there are also many emotional and mental health benefits; of particular relevance, sex without the use of condoms, culminating in ejaculation. There is also a significant body of research espousing the health benefits of the natural hormone oxytocin generated by touch, cuddles and other intimate sexual activity. The health benefits of sex for hormonally challenged women and suggestions of how to naturally increase sexual desire are included, as well as the health benefits of an open sexual lifestyle (swinging). Highlights are made of sex workers and sex surrogate assistance and how they can help keep the individual and the relationship young and vibrant. A new view on sexual health and longevity from a spiritual/energy perspective is outlined. Also included are the results of my research project, which focused on "*swingers*." The overall conclusion is that frequent sex and sexual activity can help reduce the effects of aging, keep participants healthier and feeling younger, and can benefit relationships.

INTRODUCTION

In *The Science of Orgasm* (2006), the authors refer to the World Health Organization task force meeting in Geneva 2002 for definitions of sex, sexuality and sexual health:

Sex refers to the biological characteristics of females and males but generally is used to mean "sexual activity" which includes penile-vagina-intercourse (PVI), masturbation and other ways that people exhibit their sexuality.

Sexuality encompasses sex, gender identities, sexual orientation, eroticism, pleasure, intimacy and is experienced through thoughts, fantasies, desires, beliefs, attitudes, values, behaviors, practices, roles and relationships.

Sexual health is a state of physical, emotional, mental and social well-being related to sexuality. The task force wrote: "Sexual health requires a positive and respectful approach to sexuality and sexual relationships, as well as the possibility of having pleasurable and safe sexual experiences, free of coercion, discrimination and violence."

For the purposes of my dissertation and this book, *sex* refers to orgasm via penile-vaginal-intercourse (PVI), and *other sexual activity* will refer to other aspects of lovemaking such as intimacy, cuddling, kissing, masturbation, fantasies and oral stimulation.

The studies contained herein mostly relate to heterosexual partnering as the main body of research associated with the anti-aging and health benefits of sex focuses on the beneficial effects of sexual intercourse. However, other forms of orgasm have also been shown to be beneficial, such as orgasm through masturbation, and there is a significant body of research showing the beneficial effects of cuddling and intimacy which can come from heterosexual or same sex partnering.

There have been many studies and books written about the health benefits of sex. In a white paper published by Planned Parenthood, in cooperation with the Society for the Scientific Study of Sexuality, it was pointed out that historically the belief that sex has a negative effect on the individual has been more common. Western civilization has a millennia-long tradition of sex-negative attitudes, and today's media is almost exclusively focused on the risks and dangers of sex, such as infection, addiction, abuse, pedophilia, teen pregnancy and the struggle of sexual minorities for their civil rights. However, the authors outline pioneering research that highlights the health benefits of sex, including recent studies showing how sexual activity can enhance happiness, immunity, longevity, pain management, and sexual and reproductive health.

Outlined within is the research highlighted in the White Paper and other studies including the comprehensive body of research from Stuart Brody, et al, supporting the health benefits of sex. Also included are references to a whole new realm of research into women's sexual health from a hormonal perspective.

Of particular interest are the *Anti-Aging Benefits of Sex*. Does sex and other sexual activity help halt or slow down the aging process? Does good sex help one feel younger, more youthful, and more vibrant? Is more sex the answer to not only staying young but keeping relationships young, vibrant and alive?

Anti-Aging is defined in the by the Merriam-Webster Dictionary as lessening the effects of aging or methods to preserve or extend one's lifespan. For the scientific community, anti-aging research refers to slowing, preventing, or reversing the aging process. In the medical community, anti-aging medicine means early detection, prevention, and reversal of age-related diseases. And in the wider business community, anti-aging often refers to skin care, supplements and practices that help people "look and feel younger in some way," which may have no bearing on how long people live or how healthy they actually are.

Dr. Clif Arrington, M.D., (www.anti-agingmd.com) says, "Anti-aging is any intervention intended to preserve and extend one's lifespan. All time honored health promoting behaviors such as good hygiene... diet, exercise, and stress reduction.... Current research on anti-oxidant supplementation and hormone replacement therapy is gathering evidence of 'anti-aging' activity through their ability to prevent and reverse cellular degeneration associated with aging."

There are specific educational conferences focusing on Anti-Aging Medicine, such as A4M (American Academy of Anti-Aging Medicine) that I have attended several times to find out the latest research in the field of Anti-Aging. I will include these findings as well.

I will address not only the physical benefits of sex but also the emotional, mental and spiritual health benefits of sex and other sexual activity, the anti-aging benefits of sex, the benefits of seeing sex workers and sex surrogates, and the health benefits of sexually open relationships.

My intention is to show without a doubt that more frequent sex, orgasms, and sexual activity within a partnered relationship or as a single person, does in fact slow the aging process down, increase lifespan, enhance the quality of one's health and well-being, can keep the individual feeling younger, more vibrant, and relationships can also become healthier and happier.

Note from Dr. Shelley

This research was inspired by the many individuals and couples I have worked with over the years who have complained about losing their sexual desire and were looking for ways to enhance their relationships and increase their libido. My intention was to appeal to their intellects and show them the scientific benefits of increased sexual activity so they mentally understood the benefits of increased sexual activity – inspiring them to have more sex and thus help their health and their relationships.

Chapter 1:
PHYSICAL BENEFITS OF SEX

There are many health benefits associated with sex, from pain relief to reducing the risk of breast cancer and heart disease. Surprisingly, most of the available research focuses on the maximum health benefits coming from sexual intercourse and ejaculation without condoms. There is also a significant body of research showing that fears of HIV transmission through sex without a condom may be unfounded. Infectious diseases such as herpes and other STDs are always a risk in any partnered sexual activity and it is important to be aware of these risks. It is always a personal choice whether to use condoms or not.

Many people do not have sexual partners, either because they have not found the "one," are in a sexless relationship or choose to remain single. In those situations, seeking out a "conscious sex worker," "sex surrogate," experimenting with "cougar sex," or the "swing" scene might be an option as an outlet for sexual satisfaction. In this section I will outline research on the specific physical health benefits of sex.

Note from Dr. Shelley

Ultimately a long term partner (or partners) is preferred so that the full benefits of unprotected sex can be experienced. Otherwise it is always recommended to use condoms when exploring new relationships.

Pain Relief

The medical term *prostatodynia* is characterized by urinary symptoms and pelvic pain but without signs of inflammation or infection. In a report on *prostatodynia* in 1997, Drabick et al, reported that in a United Nations peacekeeping force in Haiti the occurrence of the disorder was quite common and was associated with prolonged separation from their spouses, or lack of intercourse. Most failed to respond to multiple courses of antibiotics and masturbation had no impact, but the majority reported that resumption of normal intercourse helped relieve the symptoms.

In a study by Whipple & Komisaruk (1988), masturbation apparently led to either no improvement or to an exacerbation of pain symptoms, but vaginal stimulation, through intercourse, was shown to have substantial analgesic (pain relieving) properties, far greater than clitoral stimulation.

However, there may still be benefits from masturbation or clitoral stimulation. Ellison, in her book *Women's Sexualities* (2000), reported that orgasm may provide relief from pain. In the study, 9% of approximately 1,900 women in the United States who reported masturbating in the previous three months cited relief of menstrual cramps as their motivation.

In a report by Couch and Bearss (1990), 70% of the 82 women in their study reported having had sexual intercourse during at least 1 migraine attack. Approximately half (47%) experienced at least some relief from the headache following intercourse (17.5% reported complete relief from the headache).

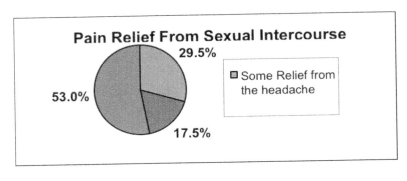

These results support the author's previous findings (1987) from a study of 34 women in which 21% reported some relief after intercourse. The research supports the hypothesis that sex and orgasms may help relieve pain.

Note from Dr. Shelley

Many of my clients have confirmed this research. It may take more effort to initiate the love-making but the benefits may well be worth it! The next time your partner complains of a headache tell them, "Studies have shown that orgasms can help reduce the pain from headaches and migraines... let's see if that's true!" Do your own research!

Vaginal and Pelvic Muscle Function

In a review of the literature on female genito–genital reflexes, Levin (2003) concluded that vaginal intercourse helps maintain vaginal and pelvic function, including penile thrusting triggering reflex muscular contractions that maintain and improve vaginal function. There were also indications that the presence of seminal component prostaglandin PGE1 in the vagina after ejaculation helps maintain vaginal oxygenation and blood flow. Improving blood flow could be expected to support sexual response and vaginal health (and perhaps general health). Using condoms, it was noted, deprives women of many benefits. It may be deduced that there are further benefits from sex than just procreation. Ejaculation may actually keep the vagina healthy.

Note from Dr. Shelley

This could be a good suggestion to make to your partner, "Research has shown that increased sexual activity can help keep you healthy 'down there' so let's make sure you get plenty!! I want to keep you healthy and happy!"

Musculoskeletal Structure:

A study by Nicholas et al (2008), examined the association of general everyday body movement with history of vaginal orgasm by asking healthy young Belgian women with known histories of either vaginal orgasm or vaginal anorgasmia (50% from each group) to be videotaped walking on the street; their vaginal orgasmic status was judged by trained (in the Functional-Sexological school) sexologists blind to their history. The gait of the vaginally orgasmic women was characterized by being physiologically normal, and manifested fluidity, energy, sensuality, freedom, and absence of both flaccid and locked muscles (greater pelvic and vertebral rotation were characteristic of the vaginally orgasmic women).

Note from Dr. Shelley

Ever noticed a sexy girl or guy walking down the street? They 'walk that walk' and turn heads. Be aware of how you strut your stuff. Be conscious of the fluidity of your movements. Sexual attractiveness comes from within, and if you are wanting to attract that special someone to you, 'walk that walk!' And if you are already in a relationship 'walking that sexy walk' can help keep the relationship young by making your partner proud to be seen out with you. Plus having more sex can help you having a more flowing, sexy walk.

Cardiovascular Health

In a study conducted from 1972 to 1975, Abramov examined the sex lives of a hundred Israeli women, aged between 40-60, who had heart attacks, compared with a control group of 100 females who had no history of heart attacks. The data showed a statistically significant correlation between frigidity (complete lack of sexual interest) and sexual dissatisfaction and between frigidity and a history of heart attack. Sexual frigidity and dissatisfaction were found among 65% of the coronary patients as compared with 24% of the controls. The same group also had an earlier menopausal age than the controls. These findings would suggest if women wish to avoid heart attacks then engaging in more sex may be the answer.

A laboratory study by Bohlem et al (2004) compared the exercise value (oxygen uptake, and blood pressure and heart rate stimulation) of men engaged in: masturbation, masturbation by a partner, and two intercourse positions (man on top and woman on top). Their results showed that intercourse produced greater duration of heart rate elevation and substantially greater oxygen uptake at orgasm than the other activities.

Note from Dr. Shelley

Another good conversation starter, "Did you know that sex is good for the heart? Research has shown that sex can keep both women's and men's hearts healthy. Maybe we should increase our sexual activity so that we can prevent heart disease!"

Prostate Cancer

An Australian study by Giles, et al (2003), of more than 2,000 men under the age of 70 who had an average of 4 or more ejaculations per week during their 20's, 30's and 40's had a significantly lower risk of developing prostate cancer than men who reported an average of less than 3 ejaculations per week.

In a US study by Leitzmann, et al (2004), at least 21 ejaculations per month was related to a decreased risk of prostate cancer in a questionnaire of more than 50,000 men between 40-75 years.

Another study by Mandel & Shuman (1987) found that compared with controls, men who had intercourse more than 3,000 times in their lives had half the risk of prostate cancer those that did not.

> **Note from Dr. Shelley**
>
> *Want more sex? Suggest to your partner that if they really want to help prevent prostrate cancer that you really should be having sex at least 3 times a week!*

Breast Cancer

A 1989 study by Lê, et al, of 51 French women who were diagnosed with breast cancer less than 3 months prior to the interview, matched with 95 controls, found increased frequency of sexual activity related to a reduced incidence of breast cancer. The higher risk of breast cancer was related with a lack of a sex partner and rare sexual intercourse (less than once a month). Women with infrequent or no intercourse had thrice the breast cancer risk of the controls (women who had more frequent sex) in the study. This could also serve to show that a long term loving relationship with regular intercourse is a good preventative measure against developing breast cancer.

> **Note from Dr. Shelley**
>
> *With breast cancer at an all time high I would suggest trying everything possible to reduce your risk! Increase your sexual activity and also your cuddle quota! Both can help reduce the risk of breast cancer. Just tell your partner, the research supports that!*

Murell, in 1995, suggested that the increased oxytocin produced during sex could be preventative in the development of breast cancer.

In a study by Rossing, et al, in 1996, women whose men used condoms or withdrawal (which generally involves the male switching from intercourse to masturbation for ejaculation), as well as women not engaging in intercourse at all, had a breast cancer rate five times higher than users of contraceptives that do not reduce vaginal exposure to semen. Greater lifetime number of sexual partners was also associated with decreased breast cancer risk, and Fraunmeni, et al (1969), found nuns to have very high rates of breast cancer.

This is in contrast to the Taoist practice in China that was popularized by Mantek Chia in his book, *Cultivating Female Sexual Energy* (1986). Chia promoted non-ejaculation as a means of helping men maintain their energy. However, scientific research, as outlined above, shows that for the purposes of reducing the risk of prostate cancer, ejaculation is important, especially for prostate health. Chia offers many great suggestions for women with regard to how to cultivate their sexual energy and I highly recommend this book for those wishing to pursue more energy aspects of cultivating their sexuality. The "Orgasmic Upward Draw" and "Microcosmic Draw" methods are definitely beneficial for internal healing and increasing and prolonging sexual pleasure.

However, as Giles (2003), Leitzmann (2004), and Mandel & Shuman (1987), have shown, the higher the frequency of ejaculations the lower the risk of prostate cancer for men, and Couch & Bearss (1990) showed the benefit of PVI and ejaculation as helping with migraine relief, and Levin (2003) outlined several benefits of women from the semen inside the vagina including increased blood flow and oxygenation.

Nutritional Content of Semen

According to Wiki.answers.com, an online source, *Semen* is an organic fluid, also known as seminal fluid. Typically, semen contains rather high nutritional content. In one typical ejaculation (approximately one teaspoon), semen contains 150 mg of protein, 11 mg of carbohydrates, 6 mg fat, 3 mg cholesterol, 7% US RDA potassium and 3% US RDA copper and zinc. There have been other studies (referred to in a study by Dissanayake, et al (2010), in the *Journal of Human Reproductive Sciences*), which show higher amounts of zinc ranging from 78.9 to 274.6 mg/L. There are trace amounts of several vitamins in a regular, healthy, ejaculation-full of semen. In fact, the amount of vitamin C is about the same as in an orange.

Semen is a natural source of proteins, vitamins, minerals and human specific components. According to www.sementherapy.com semen contains:

- ascorbic acid (vitamin C, for tissue maintenance)
- blood-group antigens (from immune system)
- calcium (mineral)
- chlorine (oxidizing agent)
- cholesterol (steroid alcohol present in body fluids)
- chlorine (base, part of the vitamin B complex)
- citric acid (occurs during cellular metabolism)
- creatine (nitrogenous substance found in muscle)
- deoxyribonucleic acid (DNA)
- fructose (sugar used for energy)
- glutathione (peptide amino acid)
- glycoproteins (cancer fighting agent)
- hyaluronidase (enzyme)
- inositol (sugar found in muscles)
- lactic acid (byproduct of muscle use)
- magnesium (mineral)
- nitrogen (gas found in all living tissue)
- phosphorus (mineral)
- prostaglandins (good for pregnancy)
- potassium (mineral)
- purine (compound of uric acid)
- pyrimidine (organic base)
- pyruvic acid (formed from either glucose or glycogen)
- selenium (cancer fighting agent)
- sodium (salt)
- sorbitol (body alcohol)
- spermidine (catalytic enzyme)
- spermine (ammonia compound found in sperm)
- urea (from urine)
- uric acid (from urine)
- vitamin B12
- zinc (mineral)

This nutritional analysis would serve to explain why Levin's study (2003), showed male ejaculate into a women's vagina results in such a transfer of life force and beneficial downstream health effects such as increased blood flow and oxygenation.

A comparison of semen by Sofikitis, et al (1993), ejaculated by the same men from masturbation and from penile-vaginal-intercourse revealed that the volume of seminal plasma, sperm count, sperm motility, and percentage of morphologically healthy sperm were all greater in the PVI samples than in the masturbation samples.

Other researchers, Purvis, et al (1986), found that compared with masturbatory samples of ejaculate, men's PVI samples had a larger semen volume and increased concentrations and total amounts of prostaglandin E and polyamines (putrescine, spermidine, and spermine). Thus, PVI involved better prostate function, larger semen volume, better quality sperm, as well as elimination of more waste products.

According to the above mentioned studies, ejaculate inside the vagina produces greater quality sperm which helps explain the enhanced health benefits for women from PVI. Ejaculate from masturbation has lesser sperm quality, although it still contains the many nutrients outlined above which could be good reason also for ingesting semen.

Note from Dr. Shelley

I know the guys will love sharing these studies about the nutritional content of semen! I actually had a vegetarian client who loved ingesting semen; she perceived it as a great source of protein! And another client shared that he increased his girlfriend's semen intake when she was pre-menstrual as the zinc component really helped balance her brain chemistry!

Concern about HIV/AIDS

Many people have concerns surrounding the risk of HIV/AIDS that comes with unprotected sexual intercourse or venturing outside of their relationship but there are several studies showing the reality of HIV and how low the risk is especially for heterosexual couples.

One of the experts on AIDS research is Stuart Brody. His research findings show that there are very few rare cases of heterosexuals getting AIDS. Apparently when the statistics are analyzed, the risk groups are intravenous drug users and people who participate in anal sex. In his book *Sex at Risk* (1997), Brody reviews nearly all the studies dealing with AIDS. Ronald Bailey in the *Wall Street Journal* review of Brody's book (December 8, 1997) says the good news is that "the risk of transmitting HIV through vaginal intercourse is nearly zero among healthy adults."

According to Mr. Brody, most scientific evidence shows that HIV is spread almost exclusively through intravenous drug use (IVDU) and receptive anal sexual intercourse (excluding infants infected in the womb, transfusion patients and hemophiliacs). And the largest study of heterosexual transmission of HIV in the U.S., undertaken by Padian, et al (1997), confirms that it is difficult for HIV to be transmitted via vaginal sex. "We estimate that infectivity for male-to-female transmission is low, approximately 0.0009% per contact, and that infectivity for female-to-male transmission is even lower." However, Dr. Padian later commented on www.AidsTruth.org, "Any attempt to refer to this or other of our publications and studies to bolster the fallacy that HIV is not transmitted heterosexually.... is a gross misrepresentation of the facts."

One study of Zambian women, by St. Lawrence, et al (2006), found that invasive medical exposures, including circumcision, were associated with greatly increased HIV incidence, but measures of sexual activity (nominally PVI, as well as lack of condom use) were not associated with increased HIV incidence or prevalence. This was also supported by further research by Deuchert & Brody (2006), and Peters, et al (2009) and their study of HIV infection in Nigeria. According to Greenhead, et al (2000), vaginal and cervical tissue could not become infected by exposure to HIV, but rectal tissue was readily infected under the same conditions.

As one research group, Dezzutti, et al (2001) noted: "Our data show that urogenital epithelial cells cannot be infected with NSI [non-syncytium-inducing] or SI [syncytium-inducing] phenotypic isolates of HIV-1" and this bench science observation was echoed by another research group, Bouschbacher, et al (2008): "HIV particles are not transmitted across the human vaginal mucosa and Langerhans cells do not increase HIV transmission." Peters, et al (2004), in their research found that PVI is associated with HIV-relevant immune benefits that were obliterated by condom use.

In summary, it seems that recent research shows that heterosexual sex between healthy adults without condoms is not as dangerous as promoted in the media. However, there are other legitimate concerns surrounding the non-use of condoms such as other sexually transmitted infections (STIs) including human papillomavirus (HPV), chlamydia, bacterial vaginosis (BV), syphilis, gonorrhea and herpes. Approximately 20 million American's have HPV and according to ww.cdc.gov, "...condoms may lower the risk of HPV. To be most effective, they should be used with every sex act, from start to finish. Condoms may also lower the risk of developing HPV-related diseases, such as genital warts and cervical cancer. But HPV can infect areas that are not covered by a condom - so condoms may not *fully* protect against HPV." And according to the same website, approximately 2.8 million chlamydia infections occur annually. It was noted that "Chlamydia can still be transmitted even if a man does not ejaculate" and is not only contracted through PVI, but can also occur with anal and oral sex. This is true of all STIs, including herpes. It is estimated that 1 in 6 people in the United States have herpes.

Long term partnered relationships where both parties have been tested for STI's would be preferable for maximizing the health benefits from PVI culminating in ejaculation. This may not always be possible, so sexual health awareness is always recommended.

Note from Dr. Shelley

Unless you know your partner's complete sexual history and trust that they have never had any other risky sexual activity or drug history it is always better to be safe than sorry. One partner may claim to have had no history with drugs, anal sex or bi-sexual activity but then their previous partners may have so until you are both tested, use condoms. Condoms do not necessarily protect you against HIV or other sexually transmitted diseases so always be aware of any cuts, lesions, or open sores and encourage honest communication.

Chapter 2:
EMOTIONAL & MENTAL BENEFITS OF SEX

There is a large body of research showing the positive health benefits of sex with regard to emotional and mental health.

In a large representative sample of the Swedish population, referred to by Brody & Costa (2009), the frequency of sexual intercourse was a significant predictor of both men's and women's greater satisfaction with their mental health. In contrast, the same study showed that masturbation was not as beneficial for mental health. The large Swedish survey also revealed that women who had experienced vaginal orgasm (defined quite conservatively as having "had an orgasm solely through the movement of the penis in the vagina") were more satisfied with their mental health than the minority of women who had only experienced orgasms through direct clitoral manipulation.

Note from Dr. Shelley

If I have gone without any sexual activity for quite some time I do start to feel a little depressed and less happy and have, on many occasions, made a conscious note of how much better I feel after having had great sex! Many of my clients and friends have also made similar comments.

Further research by Costa & Brody (2008) has shown that intercourse without a condom, culminating in orgasm, is the healthiest of all sexual activities. Not only do the studies show better mental health, but also better social interactive skills and a reduction in alexythimia (inability to perceive, identify and express emotions).

A study of Portuguese women by this same team (Brody & Costa, 2008) specifically looked at the beneficial psychological effects of sex, especially relating to those with "immature psychological defense mechanisms" – which is a term that refers to people who can't handle emotional conflict and have difficulty interacting intimately with the opposite sex, and suffer from dissociation, displacement, devaluation and isolation. In the sample of healthy Portuguese women, vaginal orgasm (triggered solely by PVI) was associated with less of the immature defenses. Brody & Costa (2009) postulate that only intercourse resulting in orgasm truly helps mental health, with regard to people with psychological issues. Brody (2009) reiterates, "It is likely that only unfettered, real PVI has important mood-enhancing benefits."

Presumably any form of orgasm would be beneficial to the health, but studies by Husted & Edwards (1976), Frohlick & Meston (2002), Cyranowski, et al (2004), and Das (2007), have shown that "higher masturbation is associated with depression" and masturbation is associated with less happiness.

One group that has both elevated rates of masturbation and of partnered sexual activities other than PVI is homosexuals. Large representative surveys, referred to by Gerressu, et al (2008), have found much higher rates of suicidal ideation, mood disorders, substance use disorders, and other psychiatric disorders in homosexual men and homosexual women than in their heterosexual counterparts (including studies conducted in what is probably one of the most pro-homosexual countries, the Netherlands, by Sandfort, et al, 2001). This tendency towards depression in homosexual men and women may also be attributed to other psychological factors such as not feeling accepted by family and society.

Another study of young women in the US, by Gallup, et al (2002), found that not only did depression test scores worsen with increasing time since last sexual intercourse but also the use of condoms obliterated the apparent antidepressant effects of PVI. Depressive symptoms and suicide attempts among women who used condoms were proportional to the consistency of condom use: more condom use means more depression and more suicide attempts.

The investigators, Burch & Gallup, suggested in a book published by Cambridge University Press (2006) that their results might be due to intravaginal absorption of seminal prostaglandins (as well as possibly seminal testosterone, luteinizing hormone [LH], and oxytocin) improving the mood of women. Even among women who rarely or never used condoms, depressive symptoms were associated with urinating after intercourse, which the investigators noted would decrease the quantity of seminal components that could be absorbed.

Perhaps one could deduce that it is advisable to hold off on urinating immediately after sex to ensure the full health benefits can be attained.

In a study by Crosby in the US (2008), compared with women who did not use condoms at all, consistent condom users were both more depressed at baseline and also evidenced a worsening of their mood during a longitudinal study.

Note from Dr. Shelley

Sex without a condom culminating in orgasm, for me, is so much more fulfilling than sex with a condom and I also find sex with another far more satisfying than masturbation. However, I do know women who can only orgasm by self masturbation and also women who have more satisfying orgasms by masturbating rather than having penile-vaginal-intercourse. Every person is different! That's what makes life and relationships interesting!

As with any research, there may be other contributing factors associated with the findings; however, this significant body of research does highlight the enhanced health benefits of sex, especially without condoms.

Better Sleep

According to Odent (1999), orgasms have a sedative effect. One study, by Ellison (2000), found that 32% of the 1,866 American women who reported masturbating in the previous 3 months did so to help them fall asleep.

Note from Dr. Shelley

It seems rather obvious that sex has a sedative effect on men – they usually fall off to sleep immediately afterwards but it is not so common with women. Many of the women I have talked with commented orgasms energize them. However, I can understand how a deeply satisfying orgasm through masturbation would help relax the person so they could fall asleep more easily. Another area for further research! Or at least a good conversation starter… "So is it true that orgasms help both men and women fall asleep? Let's try it out and see!"

Dr. Ellison conducted in-depth interviews with 70 women, ages 23-90, about sexuality, and then developed a 16-page questionnaire to survey women throughout the US. 2,632 questionnaires in total were completed. Dr. Ellison's book differentiated between goal-oriented sex and pleasure-oriented sexual experience from "outercourse" rather than "intercourse" - a term coined by Beverly Whipple and Gina Ogden.

Many of the studies outlined relating to the health benefits of sex are goal-oriented (the aim of which is orgasm in order to achieve the benefits); however, there are also many health benefits of pleasure-oriented sexual practices including the increase of oxytocin (a naturally produced hormone), which has been shown to be very important for health and well-being.

Perhaps therein lies the solution to finding health benefits from sexual activity other than intercourse? In their book, *Safe Encounters* (1989), Whipple and Ogden outline how women can say yes to pleasure and no to unsafe sex.

Oxytocin, otherwise known as the "cuddle drug" has been shown to produce many health benefits and is produced through other sexual activity or "outercourse" activities, such as kissing, holding, caressing, oral sex, thoughts, feelings, beliefs, fantasies, and dreams.

Note from Dr. Shelley

Perhaps another good ice-breaker for a potential 'date-like' situation where the two people are not really ready for the full deal (PVI) but want to explore each other sexually, or are in a new partnered situation and don't have condoms but want to experience closeness with the other... "Let's just cuddle and increase our oxytocin levels so we feel happier!"

Stress Relief

Oxytocin may also be responsible for the reduction of stress, referred to by Charnetski & Brennan (2001). The authors attribute the surge in oxytocin that accompanies sexual activity and orgasm to reduced stress. And this premise is further supported by Dr. David Weeks and Jamie James in *Secrets of the Superyoung* (1999).

Another study by Burleson, et al (2007), tracked 58 women (average age 47 years old) who recorded physical affection, several different sexual behaviors, stressful events, and mood ratings every morning for 36 weeks. The outcome of the study supports that sexual interaction and physical affection improve mood and reduce stress.

Note from Dr. Shelley

If your partner complains of being stressed from work or other life situations... suggest a cuddle session to help increase their oxytocin levels and reduce their stress levels!!

Chapter 3:
BRAIN CHEMISTRY BENEFITS OF SEX

One question that is often raised is "what if I just don't feel like it?" Many women go through perimenopause and menopause and lose interest in sex. And quite often the medical profession's response has been similar to this cartoon:

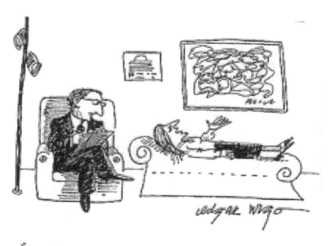

"...WHEN I TOLD HIM I'M NOT ABLE TO REACH AN ORGASM, HE SAID, 'TRY STANDING ON A CHAIR.'"

Recently however, there has been a significant increase in sexual health based medicine, especially within the Anti-Aging scientific community.

A leader in this field of Anti-Aging and Sexual Health is Dr. Sara Gottfried (www.saragottfried.com). According to Dr. Sara, "Modern women face an unacknowledged epidemic of hormonal imbalance. Unremitting stress, superwoman expectations, and misinformation about hormones have led to a full-blown crisis... We're told that it's normal to feel fatigue, anxiety ridden, unsexy, fat and cranky. *That's not true. It's not normal.*"

On orgasms helping balance the hormones, Dr. Sara writes, "Female orgasm and sexual stimulation raise estradiol levels in women who are premenopausal.... regular sexual connection and orgasm stimulate the blood flow that helps massage, soften, and thicken the tissue of the outer (vulva) and inner (vagina) pleasure equipment. Orgasm raises oxytocin, which works with estrogen in the female body to buffer stress and lower cortisol, and help women feel more connected and loving."

Note from Dr. Shelley

Menopause is often a reason women have for not wanting sex, yet there have been several studies showing the benefits of sexual activities and orgasms in helping women go through menopause! So if you or your loved one are experiencing a decrease in sexual desire and going through those menopausal changes suggest that one treatment could be having more sex and more orgasms!! All in the name of medical health benefits of course!

Dr. Ivan Rusilko (www.drivanrusilko.com), focuses on the benefits of oxytocin and how it can increase libido, decrease anxiety and reduce stress. It is often referred to as the cuddle drug and can help with intimacy and social interaction. Oxytocin, naturally produced in the body is also available as a hormonal supplement. Dr. Rusilko commented that he often prescribes it for his clients and has great success. It can help his female clients feel more loving and increase their sexual desire and can also help men with intimacy.

Dr. Lisa Tully (www.energymedicineri.com), another leader in the field of energy research, refers to oxytocin as Vitamin T (or Vitamin Touch).

Note from Dr. Shelley

For many people sometimes simply cuddling is all that is needed to satisfy them. I love cuddling, and often recommend couples to have cuddle sessions, without any further sexual activity, just simply lying in each others arms and experiencing each other. Touch is also an important aspect of intimacy that is often ignored yet so beneficial!

In their book, *A Guide to Healthy Touch: Vitamin T* (1991), Czimbal and Zadikov called Vitamin T the nurturing nutrient found in healthy touch. They write: "The US Department of Health & Happiness recommends daily doses of Vitamin T to promote growth. The main symptom of deficiency is loneliness. Natural sources of Vitamin T are handshakes, hugs, kisses, cuddles & rubs from family, friends & co-workers. Megadoses are provided by massage. Positively habit forming. Give with permission only. Guaranteed safe for all ages. Keep within reach of children. Active ingredient: TLC (tender loving care). Vitamin T is absorbed through the skin: soothes the body, calms the mind, nourishes the spirit, relieves stress, restores sense of humor, strengthens self-esteem, heals ouches (Touch minus T = ouch)."

Note from Dr. Shelley

On a trip to China I interviewed several Chinese women who complained their men did not know how to touch them, or they had never experienced loving touch, just raw, rough sex where the aim was for the man to orgasm with no emphasis on pleasure for the woman. I am sure this is also true in other countries – how sad!

Dr. Erin Lommen, another presenter at A4M, co-authored the book *Slim, Sane and Sexy* (2008) with Jay H. Mead. They discuss the old, outdated, synthetic estrogen-based hormone replacement therapy (HRT) with the newer natural bio-identical hormone replacement therapy (BHRT), for women who are experiencing hot flashes, fatigue, PMS, sleepless nights, lowered libido, and how to bring about increased energy, sexual vitality, healthy weight and a more positive outlook on life.

Note from Dr. Shelley

Hormonal testing has now become a lot more common and I always recommend any women or couples that I consult with who are experiencing a drop in libido, have difficulty sleeping, or losing weight, to get their hormonal profile done. Just recently a couple I worked with both got tested and both of them had imbalances in their hormones which when addressed resulted in such an increase of libido they felt like teenagers again! Their sexual relationship rekindled, they had more energy, lost weight and began having the best sex they had ever had, 30 years into their marriage!

Many studies have outlined the dangers of HRT with increased risk of breast, ovarian and endometrial cancer, as well as heart disease versus BHRT, which replicate the human hormones, mimicking the body's own hormone molecules in structure and action so they provide a natural boost to nudge the hormones back into balance. Referred to as "the dance of the steroids" by Dr. Lee, in his book *Natural Progesterone: The Multiple Roles of a Remarkable Hormone* (1993), Mead and Lommen in their book, said it is a continuous interactive dance between the body's sex hormones – estrogen, testosterone, and progesterone. But even bio-identical hormones, if not taken in the right balance, can cause side effects so it is essential to get accurate and reliable testing.

In chapter 5 of the *book Slim Sane and Sexy*, the authors share other dietary, herbal and life-style suggestions for improving overall health and well-being, including keeping a balanced blood sugar level by eating regularly throughout the day (every 4 ½ hours), eating a wide variety of foods, representing all the colors of the rainbow, and avoiding processed foods and refined white foods (such as baked goods made from white flour). Also, minimizing stress, slowing down, drinking more water, exercising regularly, and reducing soda pop and alcohol. They suggest choosing organic foods as much as possible to reduce the environmental pollutants on the body.

JJ Virigin has a great book, *The Virgin Diet* (2012), with specific dietary recommendations for menopausal women who want to lose weight. She suggests eliminating 7 food groups (gluten, soy, dairy, eggs, corn, peanuts, and sugar) to determine allergies and claims it is possible to lose 7 pounds in 7 days.

Note from Dr. Shelley

I did try the "Virgin" diet and lost 10 pounds over a 21 day period. Not that I was overweight but after hitting 40 those extra few pounds did sneak on. I continue not to eat gluten, soy, peanuts, corn and sugar (as much as possible), but have reintroduced some dairy and eggs. Many people have allergies to certain food groups so by cutting them out completely gives the body a chance to detox and regroup. Then reintroducing certain food groups and watching their effect on weight, energy levels and libido can be very educational! Many dairy allergies can be traced back to anti-biotic usage and the depletion of the lactose enzyme and sometimes supplementing with enzymes can help overcome those allergies. Diary foods are often very nutrient rich so eating a little is often enough.

Denie Hiestand, author of *Electrical Nutrition* (2001), specifically addresses how to increase energy levels and libido through the foods we eat and the importance of a diet low in carbohydrates (no bread, no pasta, no pizza, no cereals) and high in available protein, preferably organic sources of animal protein and animal fats.

One more leader in the field of Women's and Men's Sexual Health is Dr. Braverman. He wrote the book *Younger (sexier) You: Look and Feel 15 Years Younger by Having the Best Sex of Your Life* (2011).

Dr. Braverman states, "By keeping an active sex life, you'll feel more vibrant, smarter, more loving, and enjoy better sleep. You'll also have a greater incentive to be healthier, fitter, and thinner."

As much as we need nutritious food to live, Dr. Braverman says we need frequent and great orgasms to keep the brain and body in good health. One reason being the release of oxytocin. He suggests "3 sexual events per week for the rest of your life" as the prescription and that once a month or even once a week is not sufficient. He has a Sexual Frequency table which lists 3 times per week if you are between the ages of 40-120, 4 times if you are between 30-40, and 1 time per day if you are aged between 25-30.

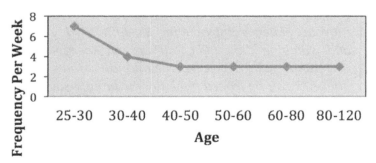

Younger (Sexier) You Sexual Frequency

Note from Dr. Shelley

Surprisingly when I mention this recommendation from Dr. Braverman, it is met with incredulous looks. In my experience not many people have a minimum of 3 sexual events per week! I aim for at least 5 per week, or more! But this could be another good conversation starter..."Did you know if you are above the age of 40 it is recommended to have sex 3 times per week? And under 30 it should be once a day? Could you possibly help me increase my quota??"

Dr. Braverman references in his book several studies outlining many health benefits of sex that back up research mentioned earlier. Sex makes you thinner - apparently you can burn up to 200 calories. It can facilitate the skin's ability to manufacture vitamin D, and oxytocin can curb the appetite and increase the loving connection; it can help the brain function quicker; reduce anxiety; help with sleep; reduce the risk of heart attack; fight infection; decrease the risk of breast cancer in women and lower the incidence of prostate cancer in men; can help relieve menstrual cramps and migraine headaches; and lead to better relationships.

Also relevant to Brain Health is a study by Brody & Preut (2002), showing ascorbic acid (vitamin C) has many functions including reduction of approach anxiety, modulation of brain dopaminergic and noradrenergic activity, cardiovascular support, oxytocin secretion, and reduction of stress. Brody refers to a double-blind randomized controlled trial of high-dose (14 days of 3,000 mg/day sustained release) ascorbic acid in healthy young German adults led to the finding that ascorbic acid caused an increase in PVI frequency, but not in frequency of masturbation or of partnered sexual behaviors other than PVI. The ascorbic acid also improved mood.

Note from Dr. Shelley

One not-so-great side-effect of increased vitamin C is that it can cause very loose bowels so don't take extra vitamin C just before you go out on a date!! Build it up slowly!!!

Akinwale (2007), studied 85 Nigerian women, aged between 50-55 years who experienced the sudden onset of sweating and/or hot flashes, associated with menopausal symptoms. 43 females were instructed to have sex at least once a week with their spouses while the other group of 42 females were instructed not to have coitus (sex). The women who had sex reported a lot lower numbers of hot flushes (41,440) or an average of 37 per week, versus the women who had no sex, who experienced a far greater number of hot flashes (141,125), or 140 per week.

The results showed a significant difference and they surmised that coitus (sex), at least once weekly lessens the frequency of hot flashes associated with menopause.

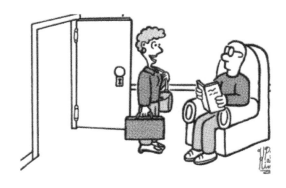

"Get naked - I need an endorphin fix."

> ### Note from Dr. Shelley
>
> *Another conversation starter... next time someone complains of hot flashes offer to help them out by giving them have a few orgasms! Or if you are a woman going through those menopausal hot flashes suggest that your partner assist you, or if you do not have a partner, this could be a great pick-up line!*

Dr. Erin Lommen, at an Anti-Aging conference in Las Vegas, shared her "DIP" theory and described what it stood for. The "D" is for the Vitamin D deficiency, the "I" for Iodine deficiency and the "P" for progesterone deficiency, which she said, is very common in menopausal women. She noted that progesterone is VERY different to progestin – the later has been attributed to an increase in breast cancer, and the former is a hormone the body naturally produces in the adrenal gland.

Progesterone depletion seems to be the norm during menopause and also iodine deficiency. According to the World Health Organization (WHO), 15 % of American women are iodine deficient and a third of the world's population is iodine deficient (*Slim, Sane and Sexy*). Environmental toxins also cause imbalances, in particular to the endocrine system, and have been linked to many major diseases ranging from cancer to Alzheimers, autism and Attention Deficit Disorder (ADD).

Another leader in this new field of Women's Sexual Health is Dr. Robyn Kutka (www.oswegopromed.com). Dr. Robyn made reference to Masters and Johnson and their *Sexual Response Cycle*, in her lecture at the A4M, and said the sexual response cycle was not relative as women are not linear. There are many different factors involved. Not only are there physiological and physical causes, but also hormonal and neurotransmitter imbalances, and lower libido due to birth control pills and anti-depressants.

Traditional skin care loaded with toxic chemicals and estrogen disruptors could also contribute to the increase in hormonal imbalance. Mr. Hiestand (author of *Electrical Nutrition* and founder of *Electric Body* healthy skincare and *theCream* natural skincare*)* is a natural health consultant. He has dedicated his life research to tracing the link to what causes dis-ease and the increase in breast cancer and other debilitating illnesses. Traditional women's skin care contains a plethora of dangerous chemicals that can be transported into the blood via daily topical application. Some of those dangerous toxins can wreck havoc on the hormones, and other toxins that the body cannot eliminate may get stored in the breast tissue and become tumors and subsequently breast cancer.

As well as looking at what we eat, drink, think and feel, it is important to also look at what we put on our skin, the body's largest absorptive organ. That is why Mr. Hiestand developed his healthy skin care, to offer women and their families truly natural alternatives to the chemically laced, and hormonally disruptive, toxin skin creams on the market.

There are many other sources linking chemicals to breast cancer, including a reference on www.medicalnewstoday.com (October, 2012), *Everyday Chemicals Raise Breast Cancer Rates.* "Ever since we have routinely added synthetic chemicals to everyday household and personal care products, the breast cancer rate among women in the UK has risen dramatically," says Breast Cancer UK, a British charity.

According to the UK office for National Statistics, in 1971 out of 100,000 women, only 66 got breast cancer; in 2010, the figure jumped to 126 per 100,000. Breast Cancer UK predicts that 1 in every 8 women will develop breast cancer at some time in their lives. A book published in 2009 titled *"No Family History"* by Sabrina McCormick, shows clearly that exposure to cosmetics, toiletries, hormones in food, and household cleaners has contributed to the increase in breast cancer rates.

Even in the neurotransmitter and hormone analysis test kit recommended by Drs. Mead and Lommen, they suggest that women restrain from using their skin care the night before they do their urinary and saliva testing as it could upset the fine hormonal balance.

Our Stolen Future, by Colborn et al, also supports this understanding of how hormonal disruptors in our environment can lead to downstream health issues that include infertility, an increase in the homosexuality and intergender population, hormonal imbalances and cancer. The greatest population implosion was noticed in alligators and frogs and it was noted that the infertility and increased occurrence of homosexuality in these species was directly related to the chemical disruptors in the environment.

Mr. Hiestand also referred to the increase in infertility due to chemical toxin overload, in one of his published articles on *The Human Race - a dying breed?* (*Healthy Options Magazine, November, 2007).* He also referred to his agricultural background growing up in New Zealand, where he noted farmers would apply topical drenches (for stomach worms, for example) directly onto the cow's skin (hide).

If chemicals can be absorbed into alligators, frogs and cows hides then it makes sense that those same environmental chemicals and hormonally disruptive toxins in skin care can also have a devastating effect, reducing libido, and altering forever our genetic makeup.

In *The Sex Researchers* (1979), Ed Brecher also connects hormonal imbalance in vitro due to chemical toxicity with gender variations in development. "In the absence of fetal androgens, the Mullerian [female] system develops and the Wolffian [male] system withers away." Too many androgens can apparently lead to a masculization of girls, and too much estrogen can lead to feminization of boys.

Dr. Lawson Wilkins referred to *The Sex Researchers,* and also studied the effects of the early progestin use on mothers and the subsequent effect on girl babies born with sexual anomalies. The synthetic progestin acted like an androgen on the female fetus that were born with signs of masculization including enlarged clitorises, and partially fused labia resembling a scrotum.

This research supports the practice of analyzing all aspects of life and living; from what is ingested, to hormonal balance, what beauty products to use, and how it can all affect sexuality, energy levels and libido.

> **Note from Dr. Shelley**
>
> *Go through you cupboards and read the labels on your beauty products, drinks and packaged food. Make healthy choices as everything affects your libido and your sexual desire. Reduce the artificial and chemical intake in your food and also in your skin care. You are ultimately responsible for you. Take action now. Make a commitment to you.*

Chapter 4:
ANTI-AGING BENEFITS OF SEX

In the introduction of his book, *Younger (sexier) You: Look and Feel 15 Years Younger by Having the Best Sex of Your Life* (2011), Dr. Braverman states: " After years of research, I've found that sex is the prescription for maintaining a youthful, abundant life." Dr. Braverman says, "Women, be ready to be sexually 30 forever. Men, be ready to be sexually 40 forever." In his opening chapter he writes, "If you could make only one change in your life to improve your chances for staying young, I'd put my money on having frequent, loving sex. Every positive sexual encounter makes your brain and body younger."

There are several studies that show the anti-aging benefits of sex, and how having sex can keep you younger. The most elaborate and detailed study was undertaken by Dr. David Weeks and Jamie James and is written up in their book *Secrets of the Superyoung.*

Weeks and James used a multimedia study, using print and electronic media, to let people know about the research and then encouraged readers or viewers to get in touch if they felt they might qualify. They received an overwhelming response and then whittled the respondents down to those that sent photos and said they looked younger, but also included those that said they felt younger. The authors emphasize, "The *superyoung* phenomena is as much a matter of *feeling* young as of *looking* younger."

They focused their research on the phenomenon of the *Superyoung* and why some people look 10 years younger than they really are. They found that people endowed with prolonged youth:

- Have more satisfying relationships, lots of great sex
- Have friendships & affairs with people 10 years younger
- Are very confident sexually
- More likely to be childless, or have smaller families
- Are extremely vigorous and athletic
- Have good posture
- Travel more widely and more often
- Have low to normal blood pressure
- Sleep deeply and well, and wake up refreshed
- Are more likely to tell the truth
- Read more and watch less TV
- Have parents who live to a healthy old age

The study consisted of the large-scale study, based upon everyone who responded, and a smaller, more intensive group of 95 people chosen from the *superyoung* in the southeast region of Scotland surrounding Edinburgh where the research group were headquartered, plus a back up control group. The researchers then did a double-blind test that used photographs to evaluate the participant's apparent age, an intensive examination of the person with questionnaires assessing their personality, attitudes towards aging, and finally a detailed face-to-face interview.

The results were very interesting, with an overwhelming majority of the *superyoung* participants looking 10-12 years younger. They all felt younger than their age, had more energy, were more resilient (were more able to bounce back from stressful, adverse life events), and adaptable (had the capacity to adjust to new situations). The authors also highlighted the importance of exercising regularly and having a "robust sex life" as being key to maintaining a youthful appearance. They state that, "Improving the quality of one's sex life can help a person to look between 4 - 7 years younger."

Another study by Palmore (1982) followed 252 racially diverse people in North Carolina over the course of 25 years. Palmore determined frequency of intercourse was a significant predictor of longevity for men. While frequency of intercourse was not predictive of longevity in women, women who reported past enjoyment of intercourse had greater longevity.

A Swedish study, by Persson (1981), of 166 seventy-year-old men, and 226 women also found an association between sexual intercourse and longevity. Five years later it was found that mortality was higher among men who had ceased having sexual intercourse at an earlier age. But no association was found with mortality for women.

Similarly, from 1979 to 1983, Davey Smith, Frankel, and Yarnell (1997), conducted a study on the relationship between frequency of orgasm and mortality in the United Kingdom. At the 10 year follow-up, they found the mortality risk was 50% lower among men who had frequent orgasms, defined in the study as two or more per week, than among men who had orgasms less than once a month.

Note from Dr. Shelley

Tell your partner you want to keep them young forever by making love to them! Or ask them, or even a stranger, to help you stay young by increasing your sexual quota!

Note from Dr. Shelley

I love meeting older, more mature people who still have a zest for life and live it to the max. I find them very sexually attractive and fascinating individuals. I definitely want to be "sexually 40 forever!" Everyone comments that I do not look my age, and I definitely don't act it! I intend to be part of the "superyoung" phenomena. I have a lot of great sex, many relationships with people 10 years or more younger than me, have a high level of sexual confidence, am very energetic, travel extensively, and have excellent health. Inspired by the movie "Harold and Maude" many years ago, I vowed to still be seducing young people (and older ones too) into life and love at the age of 80!

Chapter 5:
SPIRITUAL BENEFITS OF SEX

As well as bringing the physical, emotional and mental bodies into health and harmony, it is essential to honor our energetic and spiritual aspects.

In a recent magazine article, *Select Magazine, Jan/Feb 2013*, Deepak Chopra refers to sexual energy as the ultimate creative energy of the universe. In Ayurvedic tradition, sexual energy is recognized as a natural and vital force, and that sexual desire is a natural, powerful, and pleasurable part of who we are. Deepak Chopra says, "When you and your beloved merge physically and emotionally, you go beyond the boundaries of the ego. In this state of union, you experience timelessness, naturalness, playfulness, and defenselessness."

As Denie Hiestand, a natural health consultant and energy master, wrote in his book, *Electrical Nutrition,* "Our life-force is a subtle form of electromagnetic energy. It is the animating current of life without which we do not exist. This energy is not a recent discovery. Through the centuries, it has been called different names by many people: *light... bioplasmic energy... orgone energy... prana... chi... vital fluid... bio-cosmic energy... nature's life force...* I call it *vibrational energy,* or our *electrical life force.*" He goes on to say that this life force "flows through the body as if it were following an invisible wiring system," and this current can become weakened or partially blocked resulting in illness, physical malfunction, pain and emotional issues.

Vibrational medicine, also called energy medicine, focuses directly on the energy/electrical system to restore and reconstruct the correct electrical flow.

Caroline Myss, in her book *Anatomy of the Spirit* (1996), says, "Everything that is alive pulsates with energy and all of this energy contains information.... Your physical body is surrounded by an energy field that extends as far out as your outstretched arms and the full length of your body. It is both an information center and a highly sensitive perceptual system. We are constantly in communication with everything around us through this system, which is kind of conscious electricity that transmits and receives messages to and from other people's bodies. These messages from and within the energy field are what intuitives perceive."

Tantra, according to Wikipedia, was originally a name scholars gave to a style of religious ritual and meditation from medieval India. In the modern western world, Urban (2002), says *Tantra* has become a synonym for "spiritual sex" or "sacred sexuality" and a belief that sex is a sacred act capable of elevating its participants to a more sublime spiritual plane.

Laurie Handler, in her book *Sex & Happiness* (2007), says tantra includes practices designed to allow intense energy to circulate through the body and the ability to tune into this sexual energy, alone or with a partner, and gain more vitality and aliveness. Tantric exercises include both physical and mental meditations geared towards accelerating the practitioner to higher consciousness.

Wikipedia defines *chakras* as Indian in origin, referring to the centers of spiritual power in the human body, of which there are usually considered to be seven. According to the Tibetans, if there is an energetic imbalance in the chakras there is an almost continuous feeling of dissatisfaction, so it is essential to bring the body's energy centers into alignment.

Leadbeater's book, *The Chakras* (1927), puts forth a more modern view of the chakras, and Anodea Judith provides a fabulous "Users Guide to the Chakra System" in her book, *Wheels of Life* (1995). Judith says, "Chakras are centers of activity for the reception, assimilation and transmission of life energies."

The seven major chakras are all inseparably interrelated, and integration and balance is essential. A basic outline of the chakras is offered by Judith:

"**Chakra one**, located at the base of the spine, is associated with *survival*. Its element is *Earth*.

Chakra two, located in the lower abdomen, is associated with *emotions* and *sexuality*. Its element is *Water*.

Chakra three, located in the solar plexus, is associated with personal *power* and metabolic *energy*. Its element is *Fire*.

Chakra four, located over the sternum, is associated with *love*. Its element is *Air*.

Chakra five, located in the throat, is associated with *communication* and *creativity*. Its element is *Sound*.

Chakra six, located in the center of the forehead, is associated with *clairvoyance, intuition* and *imagination*. Its element is *Light*.

Chakra seven, located at the top of the head, is associated with *knowledge* and *understanding*. Its element is *Thought*."

There is also a school of thought that links the endocrine system with the chakras. This highlights the necessity of balancing the energy centers in order to have a balanced hormonal system.

The first chakra relates to Adrenals as they are integrally connected to our survival and are considered to be a master gland governing "fight and flight" responses. The second chakra relates to the Ovaries in women and Testes in men. The third chakra relates to the Pancreas. The fourth chakra to the Thymus. The fifth chakra to the Thyroid. The sixth chakra to the Pituitary. And the seventh chakra to the Pineal. For more information on this go to: www.healingfromtheheart.co.uk

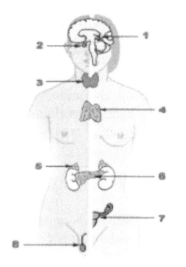

The Male and Female
Endocrine Systems

1. Pineal gland
2. Pituitary gland
3. Thyroid gland
4. Thymus
5. Adrenal gland
6. Pancreas
7. Ovary
8. Testis

(www.holisticgynps.com)

Some practices involving the balancing of the chakras/energy centers focus on meditation techniques. Other processes utilize movement, music and sexuality to activate the chakras (see: Osho Meditation Center, www.osho.com, and the *International Academy of Vibrational Wellness* trainings).

Not only are the chakras energy centers, but they can also be seen as the source of sexual energy, and blockages or issues in one chakra/energy center could result in an imbalance sexually as well as energetically.

Each chakra has a different sexual energy:

Base chakra = primal sexual urge.

Second chakra = soft and sensual loving.

Third chakra = energetic. fiery, and passionate.

Fourth chakra (heart center) = snuggling and cuddling.

Fifth chakra (throat area), = communication, talking and the noises we make (or do not make) when having sex.

Sixth chakra = connecting energetically through the sexual act, utilizing conscious breath.

Seventh chakra = ability to expand out energetically into the universe while making love.

This understanding can also be incorporated in understanding sexual health and relationships. What is it that attracts a person to a lover or partner? Perhaps when the original relationship began, the person was in a different phase of their lives, the focus was on a different chakra energy; then, as they progressed through life having families, focusing on careers, getting older, the energy may shift, and unless they are aware of these energy shifts and can bring that energy understanding to the relationship, then it could feel like the two original lovers have moved apart and are not longer connected.

As far as the sexual health of a relationship goes, understanding where each person is, with regard to their chakras and energy centers, may be helpful in the overall health of the relationship.

First it could be considered beneficial for individuals to understand their own energy system and chakras, and focus on bringing themselves into balance and harmony. And then encourage the partner to also self assess themselves. Or if the partner is not willing to look at themselves, then simply understanding where they are at "chakra wise" or energetically, can help the individual see what is needed to balance out the relationship and make it work.

The book *Soul Sex* (2004), incorporates these sexual insights about the chakras in a light-hearted story about a New Zealand girl traveling around the world in search of the ultimate sexual experience. Along the way she visits 12 different countries and activates her different chakras sexually, learning life lessons as she goes. Ultimately she realizes she wants to manifest a life partner with whom she can connect on ALL levels: sexually, physically, emotionally, mentally and spiritually.

This understanding about the chakras could be considered relevant for any counseling or therapy. Not only can this understanding of the energy centers (chakras) relate to physical symptoms manifesting in the body, emotional issues, and brain chemistry imbalances, but can also contribute to understanding the sexual body from an energetic point of view and be relevant to the overall treatment of a client's sexual issues.

Base Chakra

The base chakra is associated with the color red. It is commonly called the survival chakra and relates to those primal sexual feelings that can connect people to their bodies, root them to the earth and make their sexual survival on this earth easier. The physical developmental age frame is between 1-7 years.

When working with the base chakra, issues that may arise are experiences that occurred at birth, such as a difficult birth, or trauma around the birthing process or straight afterwards that had a physical affect on whether that energy center was compromised or allowed to fully develop. It relates physically to the sacrum, tailbone, legs and 'rootedness' in this life and in the body.

If an individual had any issues surrounding their birth and early childhood survival, quite often they may have core root sexual issues about being comfortable sexual beings, being comfortable in their raw, primal sexual expression. They may have weak constitutions; not feel comfortable sexually; not be able to truly do well on the physical plane, in their jobs, be successful making money; struggle having orgasms; or physically or sexually interacting with others.

Second Chakra

The second chakra is physically located around the pelvic area, uterus, hips, and lower back. The color associated with it is orange. The years of development in which experiences may have occurred that can detrimentally affect the development of this particular energy center and subsequent sexual energy associated with this center are from 7-14 years.

This is the time when they body develops its sexual reproductive systems and prepares for producing children later on in life. If anything occurred to inhibit the development of this energy center during those formative years, then that could lead to detrimental downstream issues physically, emotionally and sexually. There may be reproductive system issues, bad period pains, cysts, pain during sex, lower back issues, fertility issues, lower intestinal issues which could be traced back to an experience during the years of 7 to 14.

It could have been some type of physical sexual abuse, or even just a physical accident such as being kicked in the balls or landing on the bar of a bicycle. Or it could have been mentally/emotionally based such as having parents who yell and scream at their young children for being too energetic, bubbly or childlike, essentially squashing their natural development.

Third Chakra

The third chakra is physically located in the center of the body, the solar plexus, the upper intestines, the major organs such as the kidneys and liver (which process toxins). If the kidneys or liver have been compromised, that can lead to bad skin issues such as acne, eczema or psoriasis; stomach issues such as irritable bowel syndrome; empowerment issues; feeling weak, victimized, attacked; not strong emotionally, with lowered self-esteem and self-confidence. The color is associated with this energy center is yellow.

The time frame in development during which experiences can occur that can detrimentally affect the development of the third chakra is from 14-21 years. These could be considered those teenage years when there is often struggle with authority, when identity is developed, and a sense of self. It is during these years that individuals either develop into fully empowered strong sexual beings or that the energy center is compromised by events or experiences. Sexual experiences such as nonconsensual sex, being beaten up at school, judged by peers or parents for what they wear, how they do their hair, whether they can play sport or if they are considered "geeks" who prefer to read books. All of these experiences then trickle on into the individual's sexual lives – are they empowered, dominant type lovers or meek, submissive lovers?

This can also relate to the relationships people develop later in life. It can affect the sexual desires of the individual, their sexual likes and dislikes, physical issues, health issues, emotional issues, and how people relate to themselves and others, especially in relationships and sexually.

Balancing the Chakras

The ultimate achievement in this type of spiritual sexual healing is when all the energy centers (chakras) become aligned and balanced, and then it is possible for two conscious individuals to connect sexually and spiritually. Not only is it possible to connect physically, emotionally, mentally and spiritually, but also it may be possible to access heighted states of consciousness and connect to an enhanced universal reality. In my research, this is where powerful personal sexual healing can occur, and larger scale planetary healing can also transpire. The energy transmitted when two conscious souls connect sexually and orgasm in unison, can ripple out into the energetic light matrix. Ultimately, if two people connect consciously through sex then they can energetically radiate the heart frequency out into the universal consciousness and affect positive change.

This concept of energetically connecting through the physical to our light bodies and to the universal light matrix is not new. Brian Greene, in his book *The Elegant Universe* (1999), eloquently discusses the *string theory,* where "the microscopic fabric of our universe is a richly intertwined multidimensional labyrinth within which the strings of the universe endlessly twist and vibrate, rhythmically beating out the laws of the cosmos."

Donna Eden, in her book *Energy Medicine* (1998), said, "You are a latticework of energies." She encourages her readers to "Marshal these energies for your health and well being. Study your eternal dance with the unseen forces within and around you... Using the principles of energy medicine, you can optimize your body's natural capacities to heal itself and to stay healthy."

In her discussion of the chakras, she comments that sexuality may embody all seven chakras and "A sexual union where all seven chakras meet is a merging of the urge for life, the urge to create, the urge for individuality, love, expression, expanded consciousness, and spiritual union."

This is what has been called *Soul Sex*. The healing sexual energy generated can be very powerful. This type of sexual energetic understanding can be incorporated into personal growth work, and also when working with individuals and couples in a therapeutic type setting.

The more in harmony individuals become, the healthier and happier they can be in their relationships, and sex from this balanced and harmonized perspective has the possibility of having significant health and anti-aging benefits.

Note from Dr. Shelley

Bringing greater awareness to our ability to interact with ourselves or a loved one not only physically, but also emotionally, mentally, energetically and spiritually can enhance our sexual relationships. The energetic expansion that can occur is phenomenal. I encourage you as an individual to explore yourself and your energetic connections with others as it can truly expand your pleasure and enjoyment of these physical bodies and enhance your sexual experiences.

Dr. Shelley, PhD

Chapter 6:
HEALTH BENEFITS OF SEX WORKERS, SEX SURROGRATES, AND COUGAR SEX

Sex workers and Sex Surrogates

Also of interest is the use of *sex workers* and *sex surrogates* in helping individuals and couples obtain more pleasure from their sexual experiences. Sexual intercourse and good orgasms can do wonders for your health and help keep you younger. Sex can reduce your risk of prostate cancer, breast cancer, and heart disease; and can elevate your mood. If an individual has issues around intimacy or sexuality it may be advisable to visit with a *sex surrogate*. Or if the individual is not in a relationship, or in a sexless relationship, a *sex worker* may help the person explore their sexual desires and have a release for their sexual energy. Couples may also benefit from visiting with a *sex worker* as it may enhance their sex lives.

A *sex surrogate* usually refers to someone who has undergone specific training and works in tandem with a therapist, with individuals who have sexual issues.

A *sex worker* is someone who gets paid for sex.

A *conscious sex worker* refers to spiritually oriented, personal-growth escorts who provide a therapeutic session without the therapy aura. They help transform their clients with energy awareness, heart connections, touch and providing a non-judgmental atmosphere where their clients can explore their sexual fantasies in a safe setting.

Many times this type of session enables the client to maintain their home life yet find an outlet for their undealt with sexual desires. In a way these *conscious sex workers* could be seen as helping marriages stay together. This type of *conscious sex worker* session can have a very positive and powerful effect on the sexual, physical, emotional, mental and spiritual health of their clients, as well as helping to keep them young.

> **Note from Dr. Shelley**
>
> *Are you interested in learning more or enhancing your love-making skills, or spicing up your relationship? Perhaps seek out a "conscious sex worker" who can help you. For many individuals and couples this is a "safe" option as there is not the danger of emotional attachment that could come from inviting a friend or co-worker to participate. "Conscious sex workers" take their profession seriously and appreciate the opportunity to help individuals and couples experience "more."*

A *conscious sex worker* is able to perceive, with the help of their client(s), what sexual needs are not being fulfilled and help actualize those needs and meet them. It may be that the client just wants good old hard, raw sex (to meet their base chakra survival needs). It may be that they want gentle touch that they do not have in their lives (the desire for an oxytocin fix). It may be that they have such a powerful position in their jobs or are the head of the family and need to be seen as strong and powerful, yet when they come to see a *conscious sex worker* they just want to submit and lose control and be out of the drivers seat for a while to give them some respite.

Some clients want to talk about what's happening in their lives and share their feelings, their dreams, and their aspirations. Others want to go out and do things they wouldn't normally do with their partners, such as go to festivals, swing clubs, trips to exotic destination, or adventurous activities such as race car driving or sky diving. Others just want companionship or someone to have dinner with because they just want company and not to be alone. There are so many sexual needs on so many different levels and if a *sex worker* is aware they can perceive what is needed and help to create a positive experience for that client.

Many times a person seeks outside 'help' from a *sex worker* or *sex surrogate* so they can honor themselves and their needs, sexual and otherwise, helping them realize and satisfy those needs for that moment in time so that they can go back to their partners, their homes, their families and their jobs feeling better than they did and be better bosses, better partners and better parents. More often than not they also become better lovers, learning techniques they can take home to help pleasure their partners more.

Note from Dr. Shelley

I have met some amazingly conscious, empowered sex workers who truly take their profession seriously and realize that they can positively affect the individuals lives and also their relationships with their significant others. These "conscious sex workers" take pride in their work and give their heart and soul in their sessions. Often under-valued and misunderstood by society I feel it is important to acknowledge the beneficial affect these people can have in helping individuals and couples.

A *sex surrogate* is a more formal type of sex therapy work. A *sex surrogate* teaches clients sensual and sexual touch, breathing techniques, relaxation skills and sensate focus by taking them through various exercises and experiences. Most are trained and certified by the *International Professional Surrogates Association* (IPSA). *Sex surrogates* usually work with a licensed mental health professional or sex therapist and follow the ethical guidelines established by IPSA.

Sex surrogate partner therapy can be powerful and life transforming. Tamar, a well-known sex surrogate in Los Angles, outlines a lot of good information on her website: http://www.thesexsurrogate.com/

She says the clients benefit by focusing on the here and now, leaving unproductive sexual thought processes behind. Additionally, responding to the physical body helps overcome other difficulties clients may be experiencing in their lives. Leaving the talk therapy to the therapist and dealing specifically with the bodywork, the triadic relationship enables clients to positively process their experience with maximum support. Because this work is very intimate and intense, *sex surrogates* usually work with licensed psychologists, psychotherapists, Marriage and Family Therapists (MFTs) and sex therapists. Through thorough, specific support, the client receives maximum help and understanding.

The goal of the therapy is to understand and resolve whatever is inhibiting a person's sexual success so the client doesn't have to spend another day living with pain, fear or sexual discomfort.

Sex surrogates, such as Tamar, work with adults of all ages, issues and genders. On her website she lists the following as areas that she can help with:

- Reducing anxiety
- Connecting with your body's sensations
- Shedding inhibitions
- Releasing misconceptions about sex
- Learning how to ask for what you want
- Developing healthy relationships
- Feeling more comfortable with intimacy
- Addressing adult virginity
- Erectile insufficiency
- Early Ejaculation
- Delayed Ejaculation
- Shyness
- Body Image Issues
- Gaining self-love and self-acceptance
- Overcoming sexual problems
- Unlocking your unexplored sexual potential
- Developing social skills to help with dating

The movie *The Sessions* (2012), with Helen Hunt, John Hawkes and William H. Macy brought sex surrogacy into the limelight and Vena Blanchard, president of the IPSA said there is more and more of a demand for *sex surrogates*. At the present time there are approximately 50 registered sex surrogates in the US. More information sex surrogates can be found at: http://sexsurrogateofla.com

---

Note from Dr. Shelley

Sex surrogate partner therapy is very intense and I honor the people who work in this field. Sometimes talk therapy just does not do it and a physical embodiment is necessary to truly make a difference. Another hands-on therapy that is also very valuable is sexological bodywork. This type of bodywork is also achieving great results.

Cougar Sex

Another solution to the situation where a woman does not have a partner but still wants to receive the health benefits of intercourse could be to engage in *Cougar Sex*.

What is a *Cougar*? The online Urban Dictionary defines *Cougar* as, "An 'older,' experienced woman who happens to find herself in a sexual relationship with a younger man. She is not necessarily a slut, nor is she desperate. She offers sexual expertise and is open to new experiences. She simply wants to have fun. Though older, she may actually look younger than her 'hook-up.' She is attractive, confident, and just wants to have fun. She will not attempt to trap her mate into marriage, children or even an exclusive relationship. She is not interested in drama or games, as that would interfere with the pleasure she enjoys."

Usually a *Cougar* is between the ages of 40-49 and likes to seduce men 10 years younger than she is.

An early example of the *cougar* phenomenon was seen in the movie, *The Graduate,* in which middle-aged Mrs. Robinson (Ann Bancroft) seduces fresh-out-of-college Benjamin Braddock (Dustin Hoffman).

Cougar Sex can increase energy, balance the hormones, and is a great way for single women to get the health benefits of sex if they are not in a relationship. As pointed out earlier there are many wonderful health benefits associated with intercourse including pain relief; a reduction in the risk of breast cancer and heart attacks; it helps to balance hormones; and the increase in oxytocin that can result from sex can help you feel and look younger, sleep better, reduce your stress; and *cougar sex* may have other benefits too...

The Cougar

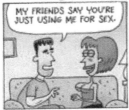 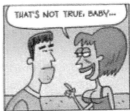 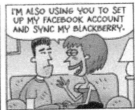

Note from Dr. Shelley

As a "cougar" myself, officially (as I am over 40), I would highly encourage women to go out "hunting!" It's fun! It is amazing how many men love it when a women is the one who makes the advances. And there are a lot of young men would relish the opportunity to be seduced by an older woman! This type of activity does not need to be limited to older, more mature women... Younger women can also benefit from going out "hunting!" I always advise any woman going out to be empowered energetically and physically. It is always good to intend a positive outcome but equally as good to be prepared. As well as carrying condoms, I recommend "Damsel in Defense" personal protection products (www.mydamselpro.net/PRO2611). They have a wide range of personal protection devices that fit easily into a small purse.

Chapter 7:
BENEFITS OF OPEN RELATIONSHIPS

As early as the 1800's, communities such as the Oneida Community on the East Coast were founded on the basis that marriage was equivalent to slavery and that no-one should 'own' another and that the true sign of enlightenment and spiritual evolvement was when a man could watch his lover being with another man and not experience jealousy.

Wolfe (2003) in her dissertation on *Jealousy and Transformation in Polyamorous Relationships*, refers to the term "compersion," which is a similar process of where one exhibits positive feelings when witnessing one's partner receiving love and erotic attention from other lovers.

> **Note from Dr. Shelley**
>
> *"Compersion" or lack of jealousy, is a fascinating concept that I have spoken and lectured on for many years. For me, it is a sign of enlightenment when one partner can watch their significant other make love with someone else and not experience jealousy but rather enjoy it. To have no fear or insecurities shows an acceptance of self and unconditional love of the other that is very rare.*

Ed Brecher, in his book *The Sex Researchers,* makes reference to this topic also, pointing out that in the larger

American culture, jealousy is expected of a spouse, whereas, "In the *swinging* subculture, the reverse is true. It is the absence of jealousy which is rewarded with praise: 'It's beautiful the way you two swing together so smoothly!'"

There are two groups in our modern society that fit this description of sexually open individuals who try to avoid jealousy and feel it more evolved to encourage openness in their relationships and sexuality. One group are those that consider themselves to be *polyamorous* (capable of loving more than one person), and the others are those involved in the *swing lifestyle*. I chose "*swingers*" as the target group for my research project.

Note from Dr. Shelley

"Polyamory" is another rarely discussed term or lifestyle choice. As a mother can love more than one child, so too, it is possible for one person to love more than one partner. As in all relationships open communication is essential and the key to the success of any relationship. As issues arise, it is important to discuss feelings and work through them. Support groups can also be very helpful and beneficial in these types of relationships.

Research Project*: Health Benefits of a Swinging Lifestyle*
Swingers can be defined as those who partake in "non-monogamous behavior in which singles or partners in a committed relationship engage in sexual activities with others as a recreational or social activity. *Swinging* can take place in a number of contexts, ranging from spontaneous sexual activity at informal gatherings of friends to planned regular social meetings, to hooking up with like-minded people at a '*swingers*' club. It can also involve Internet-based *swinger* social networking services online." (www.wikipedia.org)

I obtained my research group participants from people in the *swing* community, and received most of the answers to my survey from links I placed on a *swinger* website called: www.lifestylelounge.com.

Of particular interest were the viewpoints of *swingers* and why they participated in the *swing lifestyle*, and how their answers related to my dissertation topic of the *Anti-Aging and Health Benefits of Sex.*

I started with the basic research survey/questionnaire (which was a requirement for my Doctorate), added some specific questions at the end, then followed up with a select few for more in depth questioning.

Participating *swingers* all saw sex as an essential part of their lifestyle and relationships. The more sex they had the younger they felt, and more inspired they were to be healthier. It seems to work both ways. The healthier and sexier they felt, the more sex they wanted, and the more sex they had, the healthier and younger they felt! They all felt that having sex with others outside their main relationship benefited their relationship and increased their quality of life.

In his book *The Lifestyle* (1999), Terry Gould broke the story that **millions** of middle-class married couples in North America belonged to a worldwide subculture of *"swinging"* that the media had dismissed as a misfit relic of the 1960s.

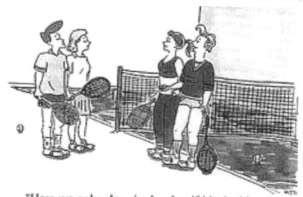

"Here we only play singles, but if it's doubles
you're interested in, come over our place tonight."

The book revealed that the vast majority of "lifestyle" couples lived conservatively in every other aspect of their lives; that there were more than 400 formally affiliated lifestyle clubs in 24 countries; that the subculture had an overseeing organization, a multimillion-dollar travel industry, and over a dozen four-star holiday resorts in Mexico and the Caribbean that catered to their needs. Large lifestyle conventions were (and still are) held a over dozen times a year in eight US states, monopolizing entire resorts for 4 days at a time, the biggest drawing 3,500 people from 437 cities in seven countries. At one Gould found, a third of the participants had post-graduate degrees, almost a third voted Republican, and forty percent considered themselves practicing Protestants, Catholics, or Jews.

These findings parallel the findings of the sample group in my Research Project. Similar to Gould's findings, the results of my research project show an overwhelming number of "educated *swingers*" – 30% had post-graduate degrees, and over 96% had college education of higher.

Over 50% said they were Catholic or Protestant, and a third considered themselves conservative politically.

Basic Demographics; Age, Gender, Education

I received a wide range of ages in the responses from 25 years old to 70 years old, however, most of the responses were from people in their 40's and the second largest group were in the 50's. Total number of responses were 166. The mean age was 48 years old (47.9).

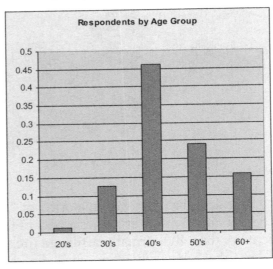

Age	Percent age
20's	1%
30's	12%
40's	48%
50's	24%
60+	15%

Perhaps this is indicative of the source of the sample for the research project. Being an online website perhaps the demographic of those that participate in such on-line sites are those in that particular age group.

Other studies of *swingers* and sexually open people such as Schubach's 1994 study showed a mean age of 46, which is quite comparable to mine. Larsen found a mean age of 39 from her 1993 data. In 2000, Cavallero, who surveyed attendees at one a national polyamory conference, found a mean age of 43, which is relatively close to the mean of my research group. And Wolfe (2003), divided her responses into male (mean age 45), and female (mean age 43), which is not too dissimilar.

I was aiming for an equal number of male *swingers* and female *swingers* but got a much greater response from male *swingers*. 75% percent of the responses were male and only 23% were females. In a total of 174 responses, 129 were from males, and 42 were female.

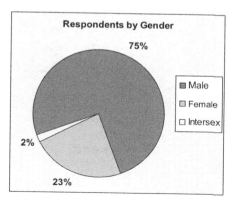

Perhaps this suggests male *swingers* are more comfortable sharing their sexual histories, or maybe it is because the female *swingers* are too busy looking after their families, working, and managing the household!

It was a predominantly white population group that responded to my survey, over 86%. The other responses consisted of 4% Black, 6% Asian/Pacific Islander, 4% Latinos, 2% Native Americans, and 1% others.

In Wolfe's 2003 research project she had an overwhelming 94.3% participants being white.

Interesting to note was the large percentage of people who had college education or higher that responded which was over 96%. This corresponds with Wolfe's research sample. 98% having received college education or higher, with 40% having graduate degrees, which is almost the same as my findings. These results parallel Loving More's 2001 survey of 1000 poly people where 96% had attended college and 40% had graduate degrees (Weber, 2002, p. 4).

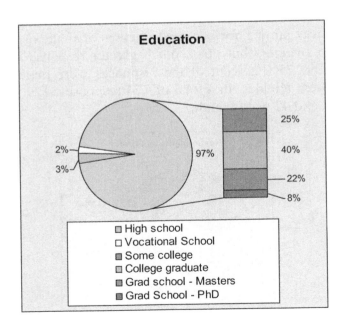

Social Demographics, Employment, Religion, Politics

A wide variety of employment was reported, including Consultants, Managers, Retired, Sales, Law, Business, Enforcement and Engineers. Plus there were a similarly wide variety of occupations for their spouses, including one "Trophy Wife."

With regard to religious affiliations, over 50% said they had a Catholic or Protestant back ground. However, over 50% responded that they never attended church, and only 32% attended once or twice a year. Only 4% attended a church service weekly. And the remaining 9% attended once a month.

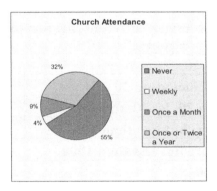

Most of the people who responded thought they were more liberal in their Political, Religious and Sexual views. Although in the Political view responses there were quite a number of people who considered themselves Conservative. This indicates that even though this group considered themselves Liberal sexually, that did not necessarily reflect their Political affiliations.

How do you think your attitudes compare with those of most people?			
Question	**More Liberal**	**Same**	**More Conservative**
Religion	68%	24%	8%
Sex	97%	2%	1%
Politics	46%	23%	32%

Sexual Experiences; Partners, Frequency, Type

In response to the question: *How Important is Sex to You*, over 95% responded that sex was considered either very important or extremely important. Over 90% reported above average to very above average sexual satisfaction.

The following question drew an interesting response: *Counting your first partner, with how many different people have you had heterosexual intercourse with, in your lifetime?* The answers ranged from 3 partners to over 2,000. Because it was a text response it was a little hard to determine statistically the results but I broke the responses down into seven groups.

With how many different people have you had heterosexual intercourse?	
Less than 10	6%
Up to and including 20	11%
More than 20, less than 50	20%
50 or more, but less than 100	22%
100 or more but less than 1000	30%
Over 1,000	2%
Lost Count or No Idea	9%

There were a total of 60 responses to this question and the average was 124 sexual partners in their lifetime (so far). The largest percentage (30%) was over 100 partners within their lifetime which is a significant increase compared with the 1993 Janus report on American sexual behavior that revealed that 60% of men and 81% of women have had fewer than 30 partners.

The results from my findings certainly seem a lot higher than those published by Mosher, Chandra, & Jones, 2005; they list males between 30-44 report an average of 6-8 female sexual partners in their lifetime and females between 30-44 report an average of 4 male sexual partners in their lifetime.

The largest and most recent is a Web-based survey conducted in fall 2005. The researchers polled a Knowledge Networks panel of 2,065 heterosexual, US non-virgins with a median age in their late 40s. The average number of sexual partners the women reported was 8.6. The average number the men reported was 31.9 (http://phys.org/news10824.html#jCp). These figures seem very low, but relate to the average American's sex life and not the average *swingers* sex life

Age of first time having sexual intercourse showed a significant amount of respondents answering 15 or less.

What was your age the first time you had sexual intercourse.	
15 or Under	28%
16 or 17	30%
18 to 21	36%
22 to 30	4%
Over 30	1%

The question: *During the past year, with how many different people have you had heterosexual intercourse*, drew answers that ranged from 1 – 300. There were a total number of 153 responses to this question, and the average was 15 sexual partners within the past year. 74% of respondents said they had between 0-10 sexual partners in the last year. This would suggest that *swingers* may not necessarily be in the lifestyle in order to get as much sex with different people as possible, but are relatively selective about who they have sex with.

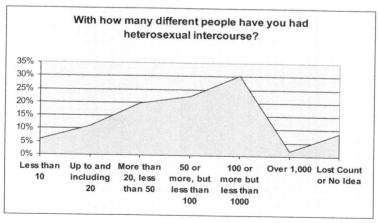

Many of the *swingers* interviewed commented that they prefer to connect at a deeper level with their swing partners and get to know them. For them, that was more rewarding. Also, if they got to know the other couples or single *swingers* then they felt more comfortable having sex without condoms and thus receiving the full health benefits of more sex.

Over 73% of *swingers* from my research project had sexual contact with someone of the same sex. On the whole *swingers* seem to be more liberal sexually. Almost 50% of the males reported having same sex sexual contact, and almost 80% of the females.

The Kinsey scale, also called the *Heterosexual-Homosexual Rating Scale*, attempts to describe a person's sexual experience and uses a scale from 0, meaning exclusively heterosexual, to 6, meaning exclusively homosexual. This scale was first published in *Sexual Behavior in the Human Male* (1948) by Alfred Kinsey, Wardell Pomeroy and others, and was also prominent in the complementary work *Sexual Behavior in the Human Female* (1953).

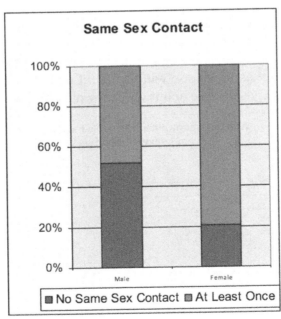

In response to the question, *"Where would you rate yourself on the Kinsey scale?"* the largest percentage of responses (37%) said they felt they would consider themselves both homosexual and heterosexual, but more heterosexual. Yet 25% self identified as exclusively heterosexual.

If we look at how people self-identify in this group of *swingers*, we find that 52% self-identified as Heterosexual and 45% as Bisexual.

Note from Dr. Shelley

Bisexuality is becoming more and more commonplace. Once again it could be indicative of a more "enlightened" spiritually evolved, less judgmental group of people who are willing to explore without limitation.

In answer to the question of whether they had ever paid a woman for sex, 41% said yes, and 59% said no. Yet, when asked whether they had ever paid a man for sex, only 7% said yes and 93% said no. This is probably indicative of the fact that over 70% of the responses to the survey came from men.

When asked if they had ever been paid for sex by a woman, 11% (17 responses) said yes, and 80% (132 responses) said no. And asked if they had ever been paid by a man for sex, 7% (11 responses) said yes, and 93% (137 reponses), said no.

There was an overwhelming response to question relating to the use of sex aids. 97% had used vibrators and 91% had used dildos. And a combined 96% said that the sex aids had been somewhat to very helpful (54% = very helpful; 42% = somewhat helpful).

Note from Dr. Shelley

Want to spice up your love life? Time to go shopping!!!! Sex toys for yourself, or for your loved one!! Have fun! Explore! See what works for you...

Health Benefits of Sex in an open relationship

In particular relevance to my doctoral dissertation were the five additional questions at the end of the survey:

1. Do you notice a change in your physical well-being after you have sex? 69% responded that they definitely noticed a positive change in their physical well-being, and 21% said they probably noticed a difference.

2. Do you notice a change in your emotional well-being after you have sex? 78% said they noticed a definite change in their emotional well-being after sex, and 17% said they probably noticed a difference.

3. Do you notice a change in your mental state after sex? 75% noticed a significant change in their mental well-being after sex, and 18% said they probably noticed a difference.

4. Do you notice you have more energy after sex? Only 43% said they definitely noticed an increase in energy after sex, 27% said probably, 17% said maybe, and 12% said probably not. This is understandable as after an expenditure of energy to achieve orgasm, sometimes there is a feeling of tiredness, predominantly in the males. And 75% of those who responded to the questionnaire were male.

5. What benefits do you feel you get from having sex? Of most relevance to my doctoral dissertation were the written responses to the question: *What benefits do you feel you get from having sex?* They were ALL positive.

As is apparent from the answers, participants in the survey felt there were many beneficial factors associated with sex. The predominance of comments related to emotional benefits, included feeling happier, more content, more pleasure, more joy; plus physical benefits included a sense of physical release, sex was seen as a form of exercise, and helped to increase energy. A large proportion also mentioned the mental benefits including stress relief, and there were also many comments about how swinging helps spouses feel closer and more in love, plus connected with others. A sense of relaxation was noted by quite a few, as was an increased spiritual connection. Plus several commented that it made them feel younger.

> ## Note from Dr. Shelley
>
> *The swingers I have met are some of the most interesting, educated, open-minded, and non-judgmental people I have ever known. Rather than stagnate within their relationships their swinging lifestyle seems to keep them young and vibrant.*

Outlined below are the comments I received *verbatim*. The responses reinforced the value and health benefits of open relationships and more sex.

Some comments were longer, such as the following:

"Morning sex leaves me with a general feeling of well-being and is a great way to kick start the day. Evening sex relaxes me and always provides a great night of sleep. Party sex with a few or several different partners is always fun, makes me feel alive, desired and gives me a lot of pleasure in both giving and receiving. It adds spice to our relationship. It is a great stress reliever. The last 2 months have been less sexually active, the stress level has been higher and now that we are upping the action again, I find that my body did not retain the always-ready mode I was used to. Perhaps a part of getting older. I know that regular sex keeps my machine well oiled, fine tuned and always ready for the road, especially as I get older! It is worth working and playing at maintaining a regular sex life for general good health and well-being"

Most of the responses simply listed several benefits in a concise way. I have grouped them into seven different categories: Physical Benefits, Emotional Benefits, Mental Benefits, Relationship Benefits, Relaxation/Stress Relief, Spiritual Benefits, Anti-Aging Benefits.

1. Physical Benefits of Open Relationships:

- *The desire to have sex inspires one to make oneself as sexually attractive as possible. This, in turn, inspires healthy activities such as exercising regularly, eating properly and generally taking care of oneself.*
- *Feeling alive, sexy, attractive and wanted.*
- *Great exercise.*
- *Feel more sexy, better about myself.*
- *Helps the heart, lungs, circulatory system, plus emotional and physical fulfillment.*
- *It is like exercise. As a personal trainer you get all the same symptoms as exercise. Increase in heart rate. Increase in body heat, creating sweat. And sometimes I am sore the next day, just like when exercising in the gym.*
- *Physical benefits of circulation, energy, aerobic activity, benefit of intimacy, confidence, feeling sexy and desirable, elevated mood, decreased stress.*
- *Cardio exercise & strengthening, lymph movement, endorphin stimulation, more relaxed, self-satisfied, self-esteem is heightened.*
- *Sex has many benefits. To name just a few, there is the physical benefits of getting one's heart rate elevated and along with the release of tension.*
- *Increased sex drive, happiness, weight-loss, a certain glow!*
- *It makes me take better care of my body.*

Note from Dr. Shelley

If you want to lose weight, rather than going to the gym (or as well as), increase your sexual quota! Suggest to your partner that it's time for some "sexercise!"

---

2. Emotional Benefits of Open Relationships:

- *The pure enjoyment of sexual pleasure with another human being. Seeing the smile on someone's face during and after while you bask in the after glow.*
- *Happy.*
- *Emotional and physical release, joy with your partner, sharing feelings and emotions, honesty, truth and Zen.*
- *Feels good, sexual satisfaction for my partner and I.*
- *I am more cheerful.*
- *Feel great.*
- *I feel satisfied, and empowered.*
- *An overall good feeling.*
- *Happier, more productive, more energy.*
- *A sense of satisfaction.*
- *Alive, healthy, happy, connected.*
- *Emotional bonding, physical relief, feeling of being wanted, feeling of belonging to human society.*

Note from Dr. Shelley

Feeling a little depressed? Perhaps it is cuddle time! Start scheduling pleasure time into your busy life!

---

3. Mental/Psychological Benefits of Open Relationships:

- *Calming of the mind and body.*
- *Mentally happier and can pay more attention to other things in life: food, water, loving, caring.*
- *Think clearer, feeling of satisfaction, not as "on edge" about other things, more feelings of being "in love and taken care of," content, happy.*
- *Mental and physical relaxation.*
- *Overall clarity and a feeling of satisfaction. I can think more clearly and stay focused on tasks.*
- *Sense of well-being, mental excitement and stimulation.*
- *Enhanced mood and mental acuity.*

Note from Dr. Shelley

Rather than a coffee break to stimulate, try a "sex break" – it may help you de-stress or think more clearly! Or next time you feel on edge or your partner is tense, suggest an orgasm or two may be the prescription!

4. Benefits for the Relationship of Open Relationships:

- *Better relationship, happier.*
- *Want to hear and accommodate my partner better.*
- *Connection with another person, mental stimulation, physical release, escape from the mundane parts of life.*
- *Interpersonal connection, physical satisfaction, emotional release.*
- *All the above especially in a swinging encounter with one or two other couples at the same time or when spouse is with another person, especially a black man, and watch her be satisfied.*
- *Gratification of my sexual needs and desires, emotional "closeness" to my partners, sense of well-being from gratifying my partners' sexual needs and desires, a sense of release.*
- *Emotional and physical bonding with my partner, release of stress.*
- *Bonding with my wife whether it be from sex with each other alone or the sex we have immediately after having sex with others.*
- *There is the feeling of intimacy with one's spouse or lover.*
- *Better relationship with my wife.*
- *Pleasure, connection with spouse, giving pleasure.*
- *Strong connection with my partner, feelings of being safe and loved by another.*
- *Shared pleasures with spouse.*
- *Brings me closer to my spouse.*
- *Feel more bonded to my spouse.*

Note from Dr. Shelley

I know many people would find it strange thinking that sharing your spouse may make you feel closer to one another but time and time again comments to that effect are expressed. Sharing with others can intensify the feelings of gratitude for your partner. It shows that you love and respect them, trust them and honor them; that their pleasure is important to you; that you love to see them happy and fulfilled; that seeing them satisfied satisfies you. This is not always the case but try it for yourself. Experiment...

---

5. Stress Relief Benefits of Open Relationships:

- *A good night sleep... cleans out my sinus's.*
- *Relaxation, better mental state of mind.*
- *I can sleep better.*
- *Satisfaction, release.*
- *More energy, less stress.*
- *Emotional connection, stress relief.*
- *Stress relief and fun.*
- *Relaxation, the ability to concentrate more clearly.*
- *Relaxation and feeling of euphoria.*
- *A more euphoric feeling and a sense of calm.*
- *Stress relief.*
- *Sexual release.*
- *Stress relief, calm relaxed feeling.*
- *Less stress, higher self esteem, higher self satisfaction, generally happier overall.*
- *Stress relief, fantasy fulfillment.*
- *As a submissive in a BDSM scene, totally spent and relaxed.*
- *Relaxed, happy, connected, desire for more sex, calm, energized, focused.*
- *Sex makes me feel complete, relaxed and energized.*
- *Physical well being, relaxation, joy, peace.*

6. Spiritual Benefits of Open Relationships:

- *Spiritual connection, relaxed, focused, clarity, balance.*
- *I feel I receive numerous benefits ranging from the physical sense stimuli to spiritual.*
- *Sex is an acknowledgment, acceptance and celebration of self and others on the most basic of levels when unfettered by religious, societal or cultural "baggage" that isn't natural to our own true being.*
- *Feeling connected to humanity. Being alive and vibrant.*
- *Freedom of expression with someone else. Connection. Energy.*

7. Anti-Aging Benefits of Open Relationships:

- *It definitely helps me feel more relaxed yet energized, happier and less bitchy, plus I feel it keeps me young.*
- *Keeps me younger.*

Summary of Research Project Findings

The group of *swingers* studied generally had a wide range of employment backgrounds; however, there were 3 times as many male respondents to females. It was fascinating to see the overwhelming number of respondents who had some college education or higher.

Respondents had a "liberal" bias towards sex and religion, but a diverse set of political beliefs. And while most respondents had religious backgrounds of being Catholic or Protestant, the majority reported not attending church at all or once or twice a year.

Respondents reported a very active sex life with multiple partners, and all respondents reported a wide range of benefits from sex, with emotional and physical benefits being reported more frequently than other benefits.

Note from Dr. Shelley

Exploring a sexually open relationship can have many benefits. Sometimes it is the wife whose libido is higher than the husband's and the husband feels good that her desires are being met, and in other scenarios it is the husband who wants to diversify with the wife's permission. There are many different types of swinging relationships where couples share with other couples - "full swap"- or where they only share with another woman, or invite a single guy to join them. Or some swinging relationships allow each individual partner to explore with or without the other partner.

Perhaps this is something you and your beloved would like to explore? Discuss it. Share your fantasies. Expand your horizons! Honest communication is key to the success of any relationship. Keep talking and sharing!

Dr. Shelley, PhD

SUMMARY

The research highlighted in this book, based on my doctoral dissertation, shows many physical health benefits associated with penile-vaginal-intercourse including reduction in pelvic pain when sexual intercourse was recommenced (Drabick; Levin); benefits to the musculoskeletal structure (Nicholas); a reduction in heart attacks (Abramov); lowered risk of prostate cancer with the greater number of ejaculations (Giles; Leitzmann; Mandel & Shuman); reduced incidence of breast cancer (Lê; Murell; Rossing); and improved blood flow and oxygenation of the vagina (Levin).

Several studies show the relative low-risk of contracting HIV/AIDS for healthy heterosexual couples that do not use condoms (Brody; Padian; St. Lawrence; Deuchert & Brody; Peters; Greenhead; Dezzutti; Boushcbacher).

Emotional and mental health benefits of sex without condoms is apparent (Brody & Costa; Gallup; Crosby). Masturbation was linked to depression (Husted & Edwards; Frohlick & Meston; Cyranowski; Das; Gerressu; Sandfort).

Oxytocin, a hormone produced during sexual activity, was shown to have several health benefits including better sleep (Odent); stress relief (Charnetski & Brennan; Weeks & James; Rusilko; Czimbal & Zadikov); mood elevation (Burleson; Brody & Preut); balancing of the hormones (Gottfried; Lommen; Braverman;); and reduction in hot flashes (Akinwale).

Hormonal imbalance and the link to chemical toxins in skincare and environmental toxins were highlighted (Colborn; Brecher; Wilkins; Kutka; Hiestand). And specific Anti-Aging benefits of sex were promoted (Braverman; Weeks).

Spiritual health and well-being in relation to sexual health and longevity was discussed, outlining the importance of balancing the chakras/energy centers. And the reference to the possible value of sex work and sex surrogates in the therapy model was made.

The findings of my basic research project focusing on *swingers* was outlined, and specific responses to questions relating to the *Anti-Aging and Health Benefits of Sex* were also summarized from the responses.

The conclusion is undeniably that sex is good for you, good for your health, helps keep you young and vibrant, keeps your relationships young, and is a necessary part of human existence.

Note from Dr. Shelley

Don't believe everything you read! Do your own research!

See if having more sex helps you with headaches or migraines. Does increased sexual activity help balance your hormones and reduce your hot flashes? Does more sex help you look and feel younger? Maybe explore the benefits of visiting a sex worker or diving into the swing scene! And have fun experimenting with energetically connecting with yourself, your partner or partners and achieving heightened states of consciousness!

Our bodies are intricate and fascinating. Relationships can be a wealth of opportunity to learn and grow. Sexual intimacy can help you, your health and well-being.

REFERENCES

Abramov, L.A. 1976. Sexual life and sexual frigidity among women developing acute myocardial infarction. *Psychosomatic Medicine 38; 6:418-425*

www.aidstruth.org/denialism/misuse/padian

Akinwale, S.O. Comparative study of coitus and non-coitus in the treatment of menopausal symptoms. *Afr J Med Med Sci 2007;36:17–21*

Atkins, R.C. *Dr. Atikins' New Diet Revolution.* New York: Avon Books, 1992.

Braverman, E.R. *Younger (sexier) You – Look and Feel 15 years Younger by Having the Best Sex of Your Life* (2011)

Bohlen, J.G., Held, J.P., Sanderson, M.O., Patterson, R.P. Heart rate, rate-pressure product, and oxygen uptake during four sexual activities. *Arch Int Med 1984;144:1745–8*

Brecher, E.M. *The Sex Researchers.* San Francisco: Specific Press, 1979.

Brody, S. Vaginal orgasm is associated with better psychological function. *Sex Relat Ther 2007;22:173–91*

Brody, S., Costa, R.M. Satisfaction (sexual, life, relationship, and mental health) is associated directly with penile-vaginal intercourse but inversely with other sexual behavior frequencies. *J Sex Med 2009;6:1947–54*

Brody, S., Costa, R.M. Vaginal orgasm is associated with less use of immature psychological defense mechanisms. *J Sex Med 2008;5:1167–76*

Brody, S. The Relative Health Benefits of Different Sexual Activities. *University of the West of Scotland, School of Social Sciences, Paisley, UK DOI: 10.1111/j.1743-6109.2009.01677.x*

Brody, S. *Sex at Risk*. New Brunswick, NY: Transaction Publishing, 1997.

Brody, S. High-dose ascorbic acid increases intercourse frequency and improves mood: A randomized controlled clinical trial. *Biol Psychiatry 2002;52:371–4*

Brody, S., Preut, R. Cannabis, tobacco, and caffeine use modify the blood pressure reactivity protection of ascorbic acid. *Pharmacol Biochem Behav 2002;72:811–6*

Brody, S., Preut, R., Schommer, K., Schurmeyer, T.H. A randomized controlled trial of high dose ascorbic acid for reduction of blood pressure, cortisol, and subjective responses to psychological stress. *Psychopharmacology 2002;159:319–24.*

Bouschbacher, M., Bomsel, M., Verronese, E., Gofflo, S., Ganor, Y., Dezutter-Dambuyant, C., Valladeau, J. Early events in HIV transmission through a human reconstructed vaginal mucosa. *AIDS 2008;22:1257–66*

Burch, R.L., Gallup, G.G.J. The psychobiology of human semen. In: Platek SM, Shackelford TK, eds. Female infidelity and paternal uncertainty: Evolutionary perspectives on male anti-cuckoldry tactics. *New York: Cambridge University Press; 2006: 141-72*

Burleson, M.H., Trevathan, W.R., & Todd, M. In the mood for love or vice versa? Exploring the relations among sexual activity, physical affection, affect, and stress in the daily lives of mid-aged women. *Arch Sex Behav. 2007 Jun; 36(3):357-68*

Charnetski, C.J., & Brennan, F. X. 2001. *Feeling Good Is Good For You: How Pleasure Can Boost Your Immune System and Lengthen Your Life.* Emmaus, PA: Rodale Press

Chia, Mantak and Chia, Maneewan. *Cultivating Female Sexual Energy.* Huntington, New York: Healing Tao Books, 1986.

Colborn, T., Dumanoski, D., and Peterson Myers, J. *Our Stolen Future (1997).*

Czimbal & Zadikov. *A Guide to Healthy Touch: Vitamin T.* Oregon: Open Book Publishers, 1991.

Costa, R.M., Brody, S. Condom use for penile-vaginal intercourse is associated with immature psychological defense mechanisms. *J Sex Med 2008;5:2522–32*

Costa, R.M., Brody, S. Immature defense mechanisms are associated with lesser vaginal orgasm consistency and greater alcohol consumption before sex. *J Sex Med 2009*

Couch, J.R., Bearss, C. Relief of migraine with sexual intercourse [abstract]. *Headache.* 1990; 30:19; 1987, 27:287.

Crosby, R., Milhausen, R., Yarber, W.L., Sanders, S.A., Graham, C.A. Condom "turn offs" among adults: An exploratory study. *Int J STD AIDS 2008;19:590–4*

Cyranowski, J.M., Bromberger, J., Youk, A., Matthews, K., Kravitz, H.M., Powell, L.H. Lifetime depression history and sexual function in women at midlife. *Arch Sex Behav 2004;33:539*

Davey Smith, G., Frankel, S., Yarnell, J. Sex and death: Are they related? Findings from the Caerphilly cohort study. *Br Med J 1997;315:1641–4*

Das, A. Masturbation in the United States. *J Sex Marital Ther, 67, 2007;33:301–17*

de Graaf, R., Sandfort, T.G., Have, M. Suicidality and sexual orientation: Differences between men and women in a general population-based sample from the Netherlands. *Arch Sex Behav 2006;35:253–62*

Deuchert, E., Brody, S. The role of health care in the spread of HIV/AIDS in Africa: Evidence from Kenya. *Int J STD AIDS 2006;17:749–52*

Dezzutti, C.S., Guenthner, P.C., Cummins, J.E. Jr., Cabrera, T., Marshall, J.H., Dillberger, A., Lal, R.B. Cervical and prostate primary epithelial cells are not productively infected but sequester human immunodeficiency virus type 1.

Dissanayake, D.M.A.B., Wijesinghe, P.S., Ratnasooriya, W.D., and Wimalasena, S. Relationship between seminal plasma zinc and semen quality in a subfertile population. *J Hum Reprod Sci. 2010 Sept-Dec; 3(3):124-128*

Drabick, J.J., Gambel, J.M., Mackey, J.F. Prostatodynia in United Nations peacekeeping forces in Haiti. *Mil Med 1997;162: 380–3.*

Ellison, C. R. *Women's Sexualities: Generations of Women Share Intimate Secrets of Sexual Self-Acceptance.* Oakland, CA: New Harbinger, 2000.

Evans, R. W. & Couch, J.R. 2001. Orgasm and migraine. *Headache 41:512-514*

Fraumeni, J.F. Jr., Lloyd, J.W., Smith, E.M., Wagoner, J.K. Cancer mortality among nuns: Role of marital status in etiology of neoplastic disease in women. *J Natl Cancer Inst 1969;42:455–68*

Frohlich, P., Meston, C. Sexual functioning and self-reported depressive symptoms among college women. *J Sex Res 2002;39:321–5*

Gallup, G.G., Burch, R.L., Platek, S.M. Does semen have antidepressant properties? *Arch Sex Behav 2002 Jun;31(3):289–93*

Gerressu, M., Mercer, C.H., Graham, C.A., Wellings, K., Johnson, A.M. Prevalence of masturbation and associated factors in a British national probability survey. *Arch Sex Behav 2008;37: 266–78*

Giles, G.G., Severi, G., English, D. R., McCredie, M.R.E., Borland, R., Boyle, P., & Hopper, J. 2003. Sexual factors and prostate cancer. *BJU International 92:211-216*

Gottfried, S. *The Hormone Cure.* New York: Scribner, 2013.

Greenhead, P., Hayes, P., Watts, P.S., Laing, K.G., Griffin, G.E., Shattock, R.J. Parameters of human immunodeficiency virus infection of human cervical tissue and inhibition by vaginal virucides. *J Virol 2000;74:5577–86*

Gould, T. *The Lifestyle.* Canada: Random House, 1999.

Handler, L. *Sex & Happiness: The Tantric Laws of Intimacy.* New York: Butterfly Workshop Press, 2007.

Hiestand, D. & S. *Electrical Nutrition.* New York: Avery/ Penguin, 2001.

Husted, J., Edwards, A. Personality correlates of male sexual arousal and behavior. *Arch Sex Behav 1976;5:149–56*

Komisaruk, B.R., Beyer-Flores, C., & Whipple, B. *The Science of Orgasm.* Baltimore: The John Hopkins University Press, 2006.

Leitzmann, M.F., Platz, E. A., Stampfer, M.J., Willett, W. C., & Giovannucci, E. 2004. Ejaculation frequency and subsequent risk of prostate cancer. *JAMA:Journal of the American Medical Association 291: 578-1586*

Lê, M.G., Bachelot, A., Hill, C. Characteristics of reproductive life and risk of breast cancer in a case-control study of young nulliparous women. *J Clin Epidemiol 1989;42:1227–33*

Leadbeater, C.W. *The Chakras.* India: Theosophical Publishing House, 1927.

Lee, J.R. *Natural Progesterone: The Multiple Roles of a Remarkable Hormone.* Sebastopol, CA: BLL Publishing, 1993.

Levin, R.J. Do women gain anything from coitus apart from pregnancy? Changes in the human female genital tract activated by coitus. *J Sex Marital Ther 2003;29:59–69*

McCormick, S. *No Family History.* New York: Rowman & Lutherfield Publishing, 2009.

Mandel JS, Schuman LM. Sexual factors and prostatic cancer: Results from a case-control study. *J Gerontol 1987;42:259–64*

Mead, J. and Lommen, E. *Slim, Sane & Sexy.* Rancho Mirage, CA: Fountain of Youth Press, 2009.

Murell, T. G. 1995. The potential for oxytocin (OT) to prevent breast cancer: a hypothesis. *Breast Cancer Research and Treatment*

35:225-229.

Myss, C. *Anatomy of the Spirit: The Seven Stages of Power and Healing.* New York: Harmony Books, 1996.

Nicholas, A., Brody, S., de Sutter, P., de Carufel, F. A woman's history of vaginal orgasm is discernible from her walk. *J Sex Med* 2008;5:2119–24

Odent, M. *The Scientification of Love.* London: Free Association Books, 1999.

Padian, N.S., Shiboski, S.C., Glass, S.O., Vittinghoff, E. Heterosexual transmission of human immunodeficiency virus (HIV) in Northern California: results from a ten-year study. *Am J Epidemiol* 1997;146:350-7

Palmore, E.B. Predictors of the longevity difference: A 25-year follow-up. *The Gerontologist 1982;22:513–8*

Pavitra, *Soul Sex: A Sexual Adventure Through the Chakras with Erotic Escapades in Exotic Lands.* Bellevue, WA: ShellDen Publishing, 2004.

Persson, G. 1981. Five-year Mortality in a 70-year-old Urban Population in Relation to Psychiatric Diagnosis Personality, Sexuality and Early Parental Death. *Acta Psychiatrica Scandinavia, 64, 244-253*

Peters, E.J., Brewer, D.D., Udonwa, N.E., Jombo, G.T.A., Essien, O.E., Umoh, V.A., Out, A.A., Eduwem, D.U., Potterat, J.J. Diverse blood exposures associated with incident HIV infection in Calabar, Nigeria. *Int J STD AIDS 2009;20:846–51*

Peters, B., Whittall, T., Babaahmady, K., Gray, K., Vaughan, R., Lehner, T. Effect of heterosexual intercourse on mucosal alloimmunisation and resistance to HIV-1 infection. *Lancet 2004;363:518–24*

Purvis, K., Magnus, O., Morkas, L., Abyholm, T., Rui, H. Ejaculate composition after masturbation and coitus in the human male. *Int J Androl 1986;9:401–6*

Rinpoche, Tenzin Wangyal, *Healing with Form, Energy, and Light.* Ithaca, New York: Snow Lion Publications, 2002.

Rossing, M.A., Stanford, J.L., Weiss, N.S., Daling, J.R. Indices of exposure to fetal and sperm antigens in relation to the occurrence of breast cancer. *Epidemiology 1996;7:309–11*

Sandfort, T.G, Bakker, F., Schellevis, F.G., Vanwesenbeeck, I. Sexual orientation and mental and physical health status: Findings from a Dutch population survey. *Am J Public Health 2006;96:1119–25*

Sandfort, T.G, de Graaf, R., Bijl, R.V, Schnabel, P. Same-sex sexual behavior and psychiatric disorders: Findings from the Netherlands Mental Health Survey and Incidence Study (NEMESIS). *Arch Gen Psychiatry 2001;58:85–91*

Sofikitis, N.V., Miyagawa, I. Endocrinological, biophysical, and biochemical parameters of semen collected via masturbation versus sexual intercourse. *J Androl 1993;14:366–73*

St. Lawrence, J.S, Klaskala, W., Kankasa, C., West, J.T., Mitchell, C.D., Wood, C. Factors associated with HIV prevalence in a pre-partum cohort of Zambian women. *Int J STD AIDS 2006;17:607–13*

Stratton, Bob & Kathy. *Swingers Guide Book (2012)*, ebook.

The Health Benefits of Sexual Expression - Planned Parenthood, 2003 (www. plannedparenthood.org)

Urban, Hugh (2002). "The Conservative Character of Tantra: Secrecy, Sacrifice and This-Worldly Power in Bengali Śākta Tantra". *International Journal of Tantric Studies* 6 (1)

Virgin, J.J. *The Virgin Diet.* Ontario, Canada: Harlequin, 2012.

Weeks, D., James, J. *Secrets of the Superyoung.* New York: Berkley Books, 1999.

Whipple, B., Komisaruk, B.R. Analgesia produced in women by genital self-stimulation. *J Sex Res 1988;24:130–40*

Whipple and Ogden. *Safe Encounters: How Women Can Say Yes to Pleasure and No to Unsafe Sex.* New York: McGraw Hill Books, 1989.

ABOUT THE AUTHOR

Dr. Shelley is a Sexologist incorporating nutrition and personal coaching into her one-to-one consulting, couples consulting, and small group workshops. She is also an international public speaker on health, well-being and sex.

One of her passions is helping women going through menopause who may have lost their sexual desire or are not happy with their relationships, body shape, or energy levels.

Dr. Shelley is also associated with a healthy skin care company called **theCream**. Their products contain no chemicals or preservatives that could disrupt the hormones or contribute to breast cancer. She is a firm believer that it is important to not only be aware of what you put in your body but also what you put on your body as the skin is the body's largest organ.

Originally from New Zealand she now lives in Las Vegas. She graduated with her PhD from the *Institute of the Advanced Study of Human Sexuality* in San Francisco, and has worked with thousands of individuals and couples over the last 20 years.

For more information visit: www.DrShelleys.com